THE LAUGHING BRAIN:

A Hierarchy of Humor by Mental
and Neural Levels

David V. Forrest, M.D.

DAVID V. FORREST M.D.

The Laughing Brain: A Hierarchy of Humor
by Mental and Neural Levels

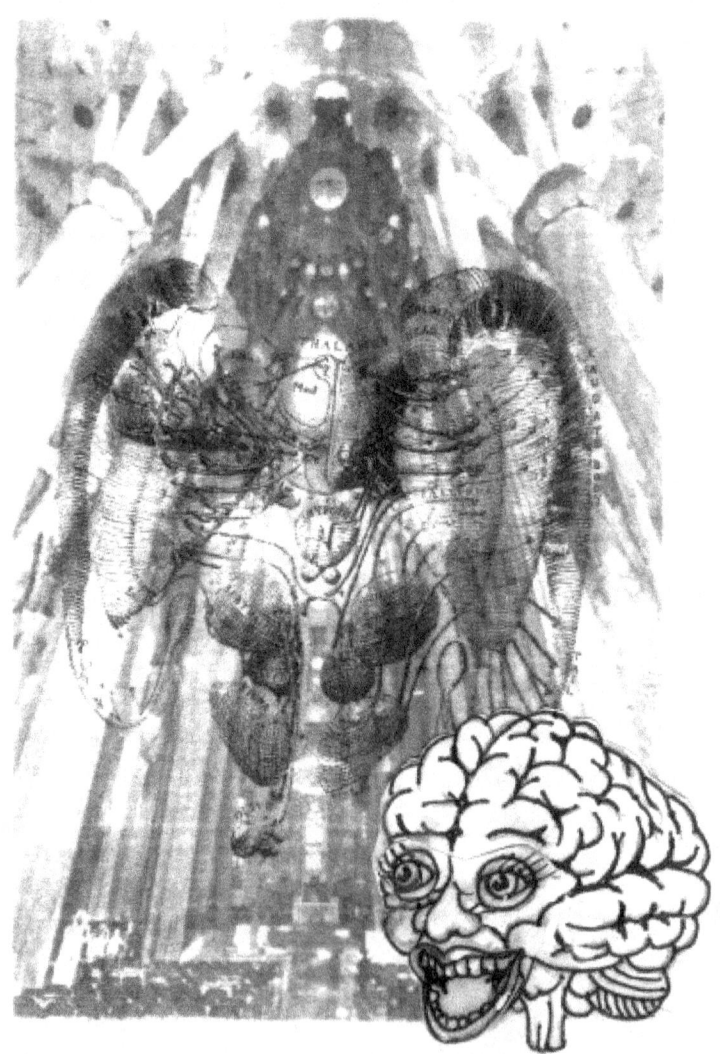

David V. Forrest, M.D.

Illustrated by the Author

Copyright 2020 David V. Forrest, M.D.

Cover image: The graceful majesty of the structures in the human brain in which motion and emotion so closely reside is superimposed upon the soaring interior of the Casa de la Sagrada Familia in Barcelona, whose elements approach living and growing bioforms, and hint at the awe that may properly be felt in contemplation of the brain's unequalled and elegant complexity.

Comments about previous books by David V. Forrest, M.D.:

Regarding *Selected American Expressions, With Street Slang Supplement, for Foreign-Born Physicians and Other Professionals,* "It is greatly appreciated by the foreign-born students and residents" -- *Medical World News*

Regarding *Slots: Praying to the God of Chance,* "In David Forrest's vision, the slot machine becomes a trope for the transcendence of desire" --Harold Bloom, Sterling Professor of English, Yale University, and author of *The American Religion*

Regarding *Beyond Eden: The Other Lives of Fine Arts Models, and the Meaning of Medical Disrobing"* -- This unique and often quite beautiful book of of portraits and interviews broaches a topic surprisingly absent from most medical school curricula: intimacy. The provocative issues raised by Dr. Forrest would profitably be addressed by physicians, who have the rare opportunity both to see their patients' bodies and hear their innermost thoughts" -- Barron Lerner, M.D., author of *The Good Doctor: A Father, A Son, and the Evolution of Medicine*

Comments about this book:

"Don't forget P.G. Wodehouse. That's pronounced 'Woodhouse'" -- John C. M. Brust, M.D., Professor of Neurology, Columbia University Vagelos College of Physicians & Surgeons

"Congratulations on a thorough treatise on humor and the brain, and your brilliant drawing skills.....In sum, this is great stuff, amazingly expansive and quite insightful....Should it have a laugh track?" -- Seth Pullman, M.D., Director, Motor Physiology Laboratory, Neurological Institute of New York

"David Forrest drills down on something I think most comedians intuitively know: what people laugh at tells us a lot about who they are and how they're doing. When someone says laughter is medicine, I now have a few footnotes to support it! Man, will I look smart! This book sits proudly on my bookshelf between Freud's *Der Witz und Seine Beziehung zum Unbewussten* and *Le Pétoman 1857-1945*" --John Lehr, comedian and actor who is the refined and offended Cave Man in Geico TV ads

"Does neuropsychiatry need comedy like a fish needs a bicycle? A read for our age of trigger warnings"--Rhonda Lieberman, author of "Glamour Wounds" in *Artforum*.

"Many thanks for your extraordinary book on humor....I will keep it as a reference and reservoir when I need some humor.' --Herbert Pardes, M.D., Executive Vice Chair of the Board of Trustees, New York-Presbyterian Hospital; Past President, American Psychiatric Association

"Dr. Forrest's book about the neurology of humor is a masterpiece" -- Blair Ford, M.D., Director, Movement Disorders Surgery Center, Director, Neurology Residency Program, Neurological Institute of New York

"Dr. Forrest introduces the concept that the human mind's response to humor is important in the diagnosis and possible treatment of various brain diseases. This is a first in-depth evaluation of this topic and starts us on the pathway of understanding both humor and brain disease, both of which are complex and not easily classified. In the end, all humor will hopefully reduce stress and have secondary positive effects on our mood as well as physiologic brain function. Read to your good health!" --Dr. Phil Stieg, Chairman of the Weill Cornell Brain and Spine Center, Neurosurgeon in Chief, New York Presbyterian Hospital, and Host, *This Is Your Brain* podcast

The Laughing Brain: A Hierarchy of Humor by Mental and Neural Levels
Ranking the Literary, Empathetic and Neurological Demands on Mind and Brain

David V. Forrest, M. D.

"Our ability to understand brain function is only as good as our understanding of the function we are studying" -- Joseph LeDoux, at Psychiatric Grand Rounds, Columbia, September 14, 2016

Dedication and Acknowledgements

This book arose from my collaboration as a psychiatrist with neurologists. It is dedicated to our patients, and to my colleagues in the Movement Disorder Group at the Neurological Institute of New York, Columbia Medical Campus, led for many years by Stanley Fahn, M.D. In addition, I gratefully acknowledge the initial encouragement and assistance of neurologist John C.M. Brust, M.D., whom I have known since he was an intern and I was a student in Medicine at Columbia; and the thoughtful suggestions of Seth Pullman, M.D. Thanks also to neurologists Lucien Côté, M.D., Serge Przedborski. M.D., Walter Nieves, M.D., Aaron Geller, M.D., Linda D. Lewis, M.D. and Karen Marder, M.D.; psychiatrists Robert Elvove, M.D., and Jeffrey Kahn, M.D.; Rhonda Lieberman, Pamela Sebastian-Ridge, Henry Case, Gordon Davis, Harry Stuart, Thalia and Philip Karajannis, Cordelia, Amy and Daniel Forrest, Matthias Karajannis, M.D., Susannah Forrest Karajannis, Paul and Adrienne Forrest, and my wife of 50 years, Lynne Stetson Forrest. My agent Glenn Hartley, and Glenn Manishin, Esq., guided me. Columbia's Departments of Psychiatry and Neurology, led by Jeffrey Lieberman, M.D. and Richard Mayeux, M.D. respectively, are fonts of lore.

Table of Contents

Introduction 9

Ranking Decisions, Three Dimensions Visualized as Three Inter-related Columns, Cognitive Operations for Humor Comprehension and Their Neural Basis, Cognitive Operations, Neural Area Correlates/Connectivity, The Creative Nature of Memory Recollection, The Various Types of Humor to Be Classified, A Unitary Dimension?, Specific Mental Faculties, Empathic Capacity, Social Awareness, Exceptions and Extenuations, Physical Empathy, Splitting the Side-Splitting, Classification of Levels of Humor, How to Use This Book/Of What Use Is This Book?, Medical Uses of This Ranking, Sensitivities and Triggers, Social Significances, Obstacles to Use in Medical Interviewing, Cultural Specificity, Evaluating Sense of Humor: A Caution, A Caveat and Invitation

The Rankings 26

Rating of 4: Social Awareness 26

High/Highbrow Humor, High Comedy, Irony/Sarcasm, Empathic Overextension, Satire, Humorous Social Observation, Repartee

Rating of 3-4: Situational Wit, Barbed Wit, Small Targets 35

Deadpan/Dry, Droll, Epigrammatic, Plays on Words, Farce, Parody, Musicality, Situational or Sitcom, High Ethnic Humor, High Gender Humor, *New Yorker* and Similar Cartoons, Women's *New Yorker* Cartoons, The Comics

Rating of 3: Something Blue 53

Blue Humor/Off Color Humor/Dirty Jokes, Limericks, Bedroom Farce/Sex Farce, Dirty Jokes, Guy Jokes

Rating of 2-3: Assassinations 58

Retributive humor, The Divine Comedy, Cynical/Sardonic Humor, Feuilleton, *Commedia dell'Arte*, Camp, Burlesque, Lampoon, Travesty, Blunder, Dark/Gallows/Morbid Humor/Black Humor/Dark Comedy/James Bond's Humor, Freud's Jokes, Jewish Comedy and Jokes, Scottish Humor, Ethnic Humor, Culture-Bound Humor, Scottish Humor, Dialect Jokes, Borscht Belt and *Schtick* Humor, Adult Animated Series, Put-Downs, Low Ethnic Humor, Light Bulb Jokes, Blond Jokes

Rating of 2: Cheaper Shots, Tasteless, Sick 77
    Caricature and Impersonation, Making Faces, Practical Joke, Low Burlesque, Sick Humor, Dead Cat/Dead Baby Jokes, Ruthless Rhymes and Little Willie, Phallic Jokes and Comedy, Dr. Strangelove Syndrome

Rating of 1-2: Unconstrained Melodies 84
    Screwball Comedy, Unintentional Humor, Spoonerisms, Freudian Slips of the Tongue, Bloopers,, Wisecracks, Shaggy Dog Stories

Rating of 1: Lowest Forms, Callow, Sophomoric, Puns 86
    Gags/One Liners/Pickup Lines, Low Comedy, Juvenile/Sophomoric, Memes for Teens and the Future of Humor, What future Humor? Children's Linguistic Prehumor, Dad Jokes, Slapstick and Sadistic Humor, Imitation of Disability, Nonsensism, Technobabble/Gobbledygook/Word Play, Doubletalk, Psychobabble, Gibbeish, Punning, Macaronic Puns, Slang and Problems of Translation, Rhyming for the Sake of Rhyming, *Klang* Associations

Rating of 0: Meaningless Hilarity 107
    Laughing at Nothing

Rating of -0.5 to -4: Nothing Funny About That 108
    Lack of a Sense of Humor, Just Kidding, Character Types Associated With a Lack of Humor

Rating of -0.5: Targets of Humor and Butts of Jokes 109
    Women According to Men

Rating of -1: Mourners and Depressed People 110

Rating of -2: Posturers 110
    (Often an Attitude Temporarily Assumed), Police Officer, Judge, Military Personnel, Political Activist Across the Political Spectrum, Sanctimonious Scold/Bluenose/Prude, Censor, Political Corrector/Language Policer, Psychiatrist or Other Therapist Who May Laugh With but Not At

Rating of -3: Zealots 111

Rating of -4: Victims and Lost Ones, Trauma, Brain Disease 111
    Dementia, Autistic Spectrum, Frontal Lobe Disease

How to Use This Ranking in Evaluations 112

Culture and Language 115
Discussion 115
Skills of the Humorist and Loci of Humor, Nature of Laughter/Gelatology, The Diaphragm, Cataplexy, Humor and the Senses, Itch and Tickling, The Cortical Homunculi and Their Representation, Smell and Taste,
Incongruity Theory, More Neural Correlations, Overview and Conclusion, *Je Ne Sais Quoi*, Emotions and Transgression in Humor, Shame and Guilt, Empathy, Kindness versus Cruelty, The Brain as a Time Organ, Robots Crack but Don't Get Jokes.

A Brief Orientation to Dementing Disorders 139
Dementia vs. Delirium, Reversible Dementias, Alzheimer's Disease, Down Syndrome, Huntington's Disease, Frontotemporal Dementia (FTD), Parkinson's Disease (PD), Parkinson Plus Syndromes: Progressive Supranuclear Palsy (PSP), Multiple System Atrophy (MSA), Corticobasal Degeneration (CBD), Diffuse Lewy Body Disease (DLB); Creuzfeldt-Jakob Disease (CJD), Chronic Traumatic Encephalopathy (CTE)/Dementia Pugilistica, Schizophrenia; Types of Protein Accumulation: Alpha-Synucleinopathies, Tauopathies, Dementias Differentiated by Frontal Lobe Function, Preserved Sense of Humor as a Socially Relevant Faculty, Cases Contrasted Regarding Preservation of Sense of Humor.

How to Speak With Patients and Their Families 155
Appendix 158
Gary Larson: Empathic Overextension/Pathetic Fallacy: Animals' Sense of Humor, Species-Specific Peculiarities, Lower Phyla, Mitochondria, Scientists, Other Sensibilities; George Booth; The Aristocrats; Imbalance, Mockery, Relationships and Unsteadiness on the Feet, The Fahn Pull Test; List of Logical Mechanisms; List of Women Comedians, The Whole Is More

References 174

THE LAUGHING BRAIN

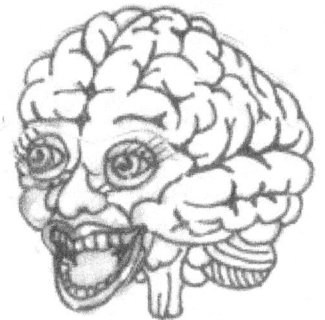

Introduction

In the November 21-22, 2015 *Wall Street Journal Review* section, an article by Susan Pinker proclaimed, "Shifts in Sense of Humor May Presage Illness," citing an article (Clark, et al. 2015) from University College London in the same month in *Journal of Alzheimer's Disease*. The study asked friends and family of patients with a type of gradually increasing dementia called frontotemporal degeneration (FTD) about any personality and behavior changes in the preceding 15 years. Regarding the patients' sense of humor, the informants noted a shift toward slapstick, satirical and absurdist humor, and also toward "darker" humor, finding mirth inappropriately in tragic events. Hysterical laughter could be brought on by everyday events others would not find funny. The authors were quoted as follows:

"As well as providing clues to underlying brain changes, subtle differences in what we find funny could help differentiate between the different diseases that cause dementia. Humor could be a particularly sensitive way of detecting dementia because it puts demands on so many different aspects of brain function, such as puzzle solving, emotion and social awareness."

Besides a general applicability in dementias, subtleties of humor are necessary for any psychiatrist's or therapist's understanding and response. I am intrigued by the possibility that deficiencies in the sense of humor may also reveal impairment of the very capacities that need be present in a therapist. Humor is a vital capability in both patient and doctor fostering therapeutic processes toward health.

Among his many helpful comments, Seth Pullman, M.D. remarked that neurologists don't usually evaluate sense of humor, because of challenges with objectivity compared with our usual mental tests, and differences in the clinicians' backgrounds and sense of humor. He added it's fun to try. If we need a number to assess and follow a patient's course (and we do), we have good tests (like the Montreal Cognitive Assessment, or

MoCA) to gauge clock drawing or spelling backwards. But if we want a feeling for a person's mind and how they relate to others, nothing beats their sense of humor.

Indeed, one hope for this ranking of humor is that it might help broaden the usually narrow conception of the dementias as just memory disorders. A person is much more than a memory. Life with even a severe memory impairment can still provide dignity and joy, depending on the integrity of other senses and faculties. Powell (2019) has suggested we are currently too focused on dementia cures that may be long in coming. A revised focus on quality of life is more reasonable for the foreseeable future, certainly for the baby boomer generation that is turning 65 at the rate of 10,000 a day. This consideration of humor in the context of dementia is not meant to imply dementia is funny. Dementia is not funny, but persons with dementia may enjoy humor at some level, just as the rest of us do. Not only does a person's sense of humor reflect what is preserved of complex higher cortical function. The sharing of humor is also a major means of affiliation. Understanding what makes a person with dementia smile or laugh can break the ice and facilitate the establishment of a connection in a person at risk of feeling lonely or shunned by acquaintances now threatened by their disability.

Ranking Decisions: Envisioning three correlated columns, I propose classifying humor by descending levels of **literary rank, cognitive and empathetic demand, and required neurological intactness**.

Douglas Hofstadter's (1979) book, *Goedel, Escher, Bach: The Eternal Golden Braid* proposed an interweaving of arts and sciences, esthetics and mathematics. and spoke of an "eternal golden braid" in conceptualizing the emergence of consciousness from recursive brain processes. Recursion allows thinking about thinking, mental movement away from the present time, and human language (Corhallis 2011). Similarly I propose the sense of humor is an interwoven braid of three mutually interacting strands that resistdisentanglement: literary subtlety, cognitive capacities and demands upon the brain. The first of my three envisioned columns ranking the literary subtlety of the types of humor will be the main focus and the spine of the scale. But first, a survey of what is involved in other two strands: the cognitive and neural dimensions.

Three Dimensions Visualized as Three Inter-related Columns:

1. **Literary levels** of types of humor from 4 down to 0 (and to -4 for degrees of humorlessness in people). Ranking these will be our organizing structure to which correspondences will be matched.

2. **Cognitive abilities/capacities/functions/operations** needed for (1)

3. **Neurological integrity/intactness** required for (1) and (2)

Cognitive Operations for Humor Comprehension and Their Neural Basis:

Chan et al (2015) outlined the cognitive operations in 'getting a joke,' which always requires resolving an incongruity, whether it be bridging an inference, exaggeration, or ambiguity. To be 'gotten', all jokes require integrity of the dorsolateral prefrontal cortex for script shifting, which I would add is a function of working memory--holding and processing mental elements. Thus jokes and much other humor involve a **bait and switch** manipulation and an element of **surprise.** In the set up, the joke teller leads the hearer down one path, then abruptly moves them to another at the punch line. much like the *reveal* at the end of a magic trick. The intact hearer may laugh or groan at being taken or slightly suckered. If the working memory and other executive function is not intact, a person may *perseverate,* that is, become stuck in the initial mental set and fail to move on to the following thought, especially if it catches them by surprise or requires also a shift in the level of abstraction or metaphor. The ventral anterior cingulate cortex is involved in the actual 'getting' and affective appreciation. Other areas include the temporo-parietal cortex for theory of mind, or mind-mindfulness; and the fronto-parietal cortex for executive retrieval from memory, awareness of oneself, and interpretation of language. The orbitofrontal cortex, amygdala and parahippocampal gyrus support social and emotional aspects of humor.

On a purely neuroanatomic basis, at least part of the metaphorical 'funny bone'-sense of humor- has been located, and it is in the cingulum. Bijanki et al. (2019) stimulated the left dorsal anterior cingulum bundle in 3 awake neurosurgery patients with epilepsy, and found both decreased anxiety (anxiolysis) and a positive, mirthful affect resulted.

Anjan Chatterjee (Pierce, 2015) traced a the brain path of a simple joke, e.g.: "I went to buy camouflage pants but couldn't find any." The prefrontal cortex assembles the elements, the cingulate cortex detects error, in this case ambiguity, that is the exaggeration that the pants were so camouflaged they weren't findable, and amusement arises in temporo-parietal areas in connection with the limbic amygdala, and this activates the reward center (the nucleus accumbens) with a shot of dopamine. There is an 'ah-hah' surprise element, and respiratory centers activate a laugh (the term 'ah-hah' even sounds respiratory). To summarize, operationally:

Cognitive Operations in 5 Steps
1. Detect exaggeration/comparison/distortion/
incongruity/disparity

Example: Charles Shultz's comic child Charlie Brown in a cartoon consulting his elder sister Lucy, who has set up shop to give "Psychiatric Help 5 cents, Summer Rate 4 cents." Lucy tells Charlie, "You are pathetic and will be alone forever! Now pay me my 5 cents!"

Example: Drawing of the Pentagon with a giant roulette wheel in its courtyard, exaggerating an apprehension that a Commander in Chief who emerged from the casino industry might be a gamble (author's cartoon, 2016).

Figure: Pentagon roulette

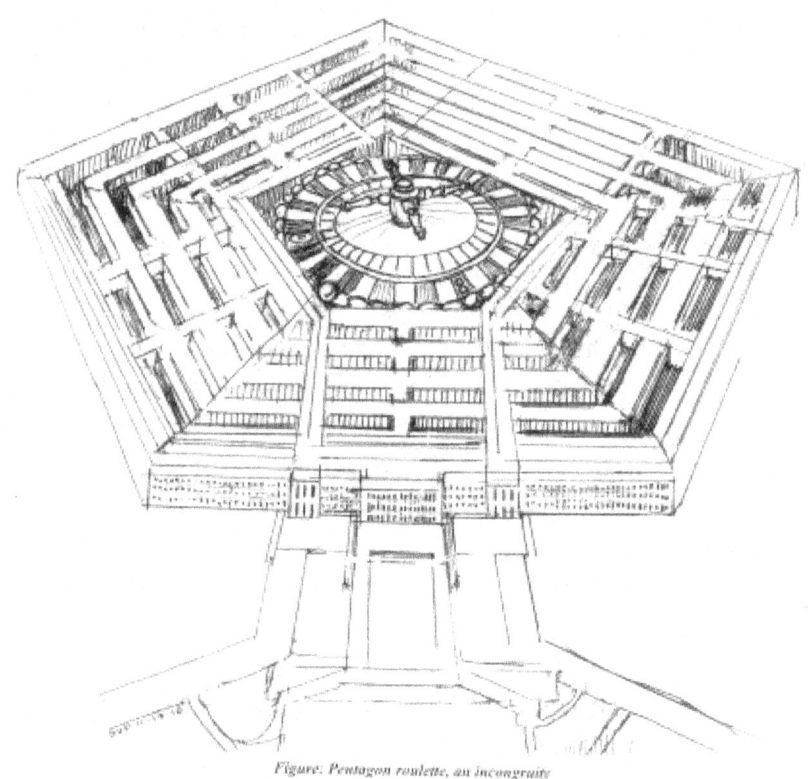

Figure: Pentagon roulette, an incongruity

In the Pentagon cartoon, which was drawn on November 19, 2016 just after the Presidential election, a giant roulette wheel is impossibly superimposed upon the Pentagon to express apprehension that a Commander in Chief who emerged from the casino industry might prove chancy. The tasks of the Presidency, comprehending and acting in a complex world are daunting, and perhaps more so for one who avoided serving, even granted his having had some military schooling. On November 17, 2018 the not-too-Trump-friendly New York Times *featured an opinion piece by Helene Cooper and others (2018) entitled "2 Years In, Still Struggling to Understand 'My Military.'"* Baker (2019) in an essay, "The Strangely Dovish Donald Trump," proposed that "Trump seems to be genuinely trying to tilt the U.S. security posture away from the ready projection of force that has been a defining feature...." But on January 3, 2020, following the storming of our embassy, he did blow Soleimani away. He has declared himself a "wartime President" against COVID-19.

This cartoon broadly illustrates the comparative essence of humor, whether it exaggerates its subject to a funny extent, or contrasts behavior with a social standard; or in this case, amalgamates incongruous things that don't belong together. Dr. Samuel Johnson (On Metaphysical Wit, 1779) similarly said of the Metaphysical poetry movement, "the most heterogeneous ideas are yoked by violence together." Both poetry and humor freely do this.

Example: The comic Amy Schumer appearing on the Ellen DeGeneres daytime show (8 February 2018) in toddlers' clothes to poke fun at the cult of youth.

Example: A *New Yorker* cartoon (August 6-13, 2018) of two men in hazmat suits contemplating an open pizza box in which the three remaining slices have formed the ionizing radiation warning symbol (the trefoil).

Example: An October 2018 ad for Geico insurance depicting NFL Minnesota Vikings wide receiver Stefon Diggs attempting to take out the trash, while one man says to another, "I can't believe how everything sticks to Stefon's hands." As the trash and even the trash can stick to Stefan's hands, one of the men says, "He plays football, doesn't he?"

Example: Drawing of two musicians dueling with triangles.

Figure: Dueling triangles

Incongruity is a basic component of humor recognized even by babies. Dueling musical instruments are incongruous as they are not weapons but instruments of usually blissful musical performance. Thus dueling violins, dueling cellos and dueling pianos have recently entertained and, in the case of my young sports-minded grandson, even inspired taking up the violin (furiously). One form of incongruity is disparity. This cartoon plays with the incongruity of dueling instruments, and adds the disparity of the
instrument being the triangle, which is a still less mighty dueling weapon and also funny, my 11-year-old violinist grandson says, because it can only play one note.

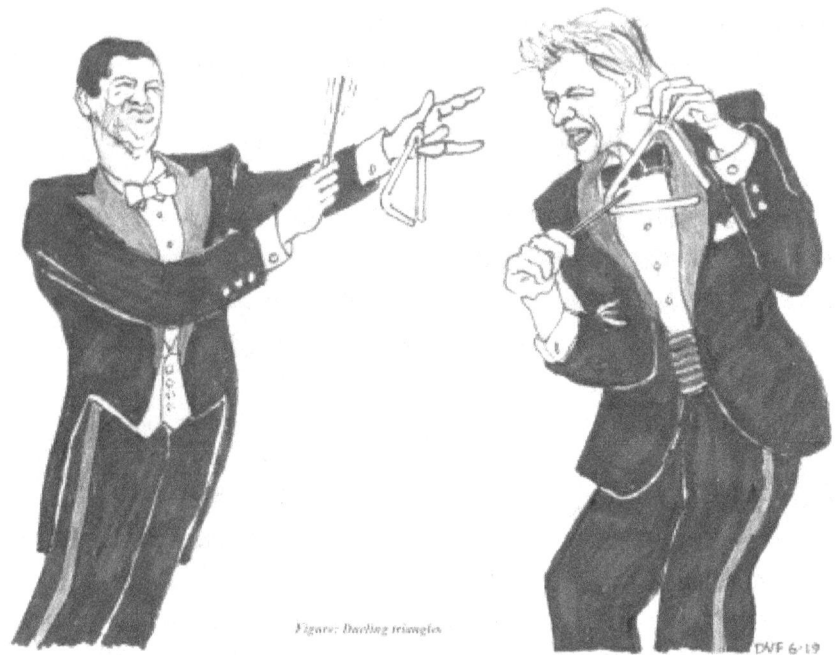

Figure: Dueling triangles

Similarly, there was a 2019 Geico insurance TV ad in which a musician kept hitting his triangle while cavorting like a rock star back and forth on the stage in front of the orchestra, while the announcer intoned, "A triangle solo is surprising. What's not surprising is how much you save on car insurance with Geico."

Terry Eagelton (2019a, 2019b) relates many theories of humor to incongruity, though he mentions a release of tension (analogous even to sexual climax) and a way to feel superior (like *schadenfreude* or targeting), which we shall consider lower in the rankings.

OK, now returning to the 5 Cognitive Steps:
1. Detect incongruity/disparity as in above examples
2. Match against actual

Assess discrepancy (this is already present in a 12-18 month infant); the Ah-ha! of getting the joke, as in examples:

To belabor the obvious, needless I hope to say, unlike Lucy in the example, above, we real psychiatrists help patients feel better, not condemn them to perpetual loneliness. There is

no giant roulette wheel at the Pentagon, Amy Schumer is past toddlerhood, pizza slices aren't a hazard sign, and while Stefon Diggs is very good at catching footballs, it isn't because his hands are so sticky that all things stick to them.
3. Empathize, be touched, involved, as much as capable of this
4. Identify with target of humor, yet keep observer's distance
5. Release laughter, as deeper feelings emerge or explode.

Neural Area Correlates and Connectivity: Some assembly is required, to link up the sequence of connected brain regions:
1. Afferent (sensory) inputs (intact hearing, vision. etc)
2. Cortical centers for recognition of language, images, actions (based on learned experience)
3. Dorsolateral prefrontal cortex for executive assembly
4. Left frontal lobe for simple, right frontal lobe for complex and externally generated components
5. Specialized areas, e.g. fusiform (occipitotemporal) gyrus (facial recognition), right posterior superior temporal sulcus (facial emotion), temporo-parietal junction (self-other distinctions, theory of mind, moral decisions, out-of-body experiences when impaired), parietal lobe (spatiality), cerebellum, basal ganglia motor areas (proprioceptive capability, getting physical humor)
6. Cingulate gyrus to "get" joke (comparison, valuation)
7. Amygdala for emotional loading
8. Respiratory centers for laughter.

The Creative Nature of Memory Re-collection

Given that a ranking of humor is relevant to degrees and types of dementia, the nature of memory needs explaining. **Dementia** is much more than remembering, involving also comprehension, processing, comparison, abstraction, and empathy among other functions. But remembering itself is complex, and not rote data entry. First of all, **registration** means receiving and recording a memory. Many, perhaps most patients thought to have trouble with memory **retrieval** are having interference with registration caused by other disorders or side effects. But once the traces from the outside world arrive from the sense organs to the hippocampus, the process has just begun. Nothing is engraved upon the hippocampus, which passes memory traces on like hot potatoes to areas of the cerebral cortex. Get KO'ed during this 20-minute process and you'll have retrograde amnesia for the whole 20 minutes. Laying down a long-term memory is not fully understood, but it involves comparisons with what is already stored and it involves breaking down the content into elements and sending them to separate, specialized areas of the brain. Remembering reverses the process. It literally *re-collects* the elements from their specialized storage and re-assembles them into what feels like the original impression. Again, "some assembly required" is the nature of recall. As you may suspect. this "game of telephone" in the brain introduces distortions and errors. Remembering is creative in that it amalgamates other similar traces, cross-talk from other memories, wishful emotional inputs and conceptual preconceptions. Mnemonists rely on associative strings and webs, and people with "middle-age forgetting," which is not considered dementia, will easier forget isolated data points like a name or a number than song lyrics or a spouse's food preferences imbedded in many experiences. Explicit or declarative memories for factoids are also easier to misplace than implicit memories like riding a bike or typing or cooking or drawing, or the feelings we have about people. The brain also has specialized cubbyholes for certain categories of memories like faces or learned languages.

Much is known about the odd categories of our memory traces, which may be according to purpose or use. I heard of a pet cat who liked to line up his toys and, upon killing a mouse, added it to his line of things for play use.

As an indication of the complex, constructed, and emotional nature of memory, think of the unreliability of eyewitnesses. Memory is a hodge-podge of amalgamated and overlapping sources, what psychiatrists and analysts term overedetermination, and our desires enter in..

Memory disorders need to be judged in the light of the fraught nature of normal remembering processes.

The Various Types of Humor to Be Classified

Different forms of humor are listed in dictionaries of literary terms (Shaw 1972, Cuddon 1976) which, being alphabetical, are not ranked in a hierarchical way.

What is needed for various uses is a classification of the subtleties of humor according to the cognitive capacity each level requires, described as mental functions. These levels of higher cortical functions can then be correlated in neuropsychiatry with the intactness of levels of the neuraxis they require. In clinical application, changes in the patient's level of humor can tactfully be explored with the patient and family. What stimuli provoke laughter can be noted along with changes in reading and viewing habits. Patients and informants have little trouble telling what is laughed at.

A Unitary Dimension?

Does it make sense to construct a hierarchy in a single dimension? There are lacks or failures of **specific mental faculties**. Problems in these agencies might weigh against a single linear ranking. Obvious examples would be impairments of the senses necessary to apprehend types of humor, such as blindness, ocular or cortical; and deafness, of conduction or nerve origin. But these can often be circumvented so appreciation of humor can remain intact.

Other impairments may eliminate a type of humor in an otherwise intact individual. For example, prosopagnosia, the absence of ability to recognize faces, could obviate appreciation of caricature or impersonation. Oliver Sacks, who had prosopagnosia, retained a sense of humor otherwise, as all of us who knew him can attest.

Should **empathic capacity** have its own dimension? Empathy is so important to higher levels of humor that I single it out first for consideration. It is impaired in persons with some dementias, especially frontotemporal, in those on the autistic spectrum, and in many with severe sociopathy or addiction who may possess conceptual competence but lack a social conscience. Suffering chronic pain may also impair empathy, and so do some degenerative neurological disorders, as we shall discuss later. Montgomery Clift, in a triumph of acting, which requires empathic projective identification, returned to shooting the 1956 film *Raintree County* in severe pain from an auto accident only 2 months earlier. Rather astonishingly, a Yale psychologist (Bloom, 2016) has railed against empathy as too feeling, and suggested a more removed, thoughtful and less focused "rational compassion" that relies on rules and principles as a fairer virtue, and less biased, because it does not require us to select persons like us to see as ourselves. George Bernard Shaw once defined compassion as the fellow-feeling of the unsound, to which I would rejoin, who of us is sound? Compassion is a more patronizing stance than empathy, which humbly and emotionally admits our common human condition.

Social awareness could be its own dimension. Developing it depends on interpersonal and social experience. Good-enough parenting and skin-to-skin touch is vital to child development, as deprivation studies have shown. Social awareness and an appreciation of what is universal to the human experience are part of the highest level of humor. The French philosopher Henri Bergson thought the essence of the humorous was deviation from social expectations, whether intentionally or unintentionally non-conforming.

Exceptions and extenuations aside, I prefer to remain with a linear hierarchy, because those possible other lines are essential ingredients of what is high and low, together with such humor-appreciating abilities as verbal and visual skills, abstracting ability, supra-span memory and attention span. Even visual spatial abilities can come to play in appreciating physical comedy, as in Jerome Robbins's spoof ballet, *The Concert,* or the pratfalls of Charlie Chaplain, Jerry Lewis and Chevy Chase. This capacity might be called **Physical Empathy**, discussed under **Slapstick**.

Splitting the Side-Splitting

To begin with the classification, the following is an attempt to rate types of humor according to what they require in cognitive, empathic and all other demands, on a 0-4 scale in which 4 is the most demanding. In medicine we often rate from 0-4 (although there are 5 levels of kidney failure, for example), but I opted for intermediate levels and added a minus scale of -1 to -4 for lacking a sense of humor. At the zero and minus levels, I shall move freely from ranking qualities of the comedic stimulus to ranking the receptive mindsets of individuals who react (or choose not to react or fail to react) at those levels.

Classification of Levels of Humor

The scale begins at the top, that is, humor that demands the highest esthetic appreciation, cognitive capacity and neurological integrity. Humor that warrants this ranking manifests social awareness and commentary, embraces all humankind, and includes empathy. Encapsulating universal and unusually deep insights, it is not limited by narrowly self-reflective, group-oriented or culture bound ingredients, and is often emotionally complex. Thus the demands of the highest level of humor, that require fully intact appreciation (here proposed) are:

1. Social awareness vs. self-centered
2. Universal vision beyond self or group
3. Emotional empathy vs. unfeeling distance or cruelty
4. Metaphorical/abstracting capability vs. concreteness, literalness; associations necessary for comparisons
5. Verbal intelligence (images, sounds for word play)
6. Visual sensibility (for humor in art, cartoons, memes)
7. Facial emotion recognition, also voice tone, timing.
8. Physical/gestural, proprioceptive receptiveness and bodily awareness (for physical humor).

How to Use this Book/Of What Use Is This Book?

Humor in its many aspects is of broad cultural interest and it is critical to understanding one another and to our well-being. I have found the levels of humor to be an intriguing conversational subject for many people, even at the dinner table. Folks are happy to provide examples of what they find funny, and what people they know find funny. Some argue about the ranking of certain comedy or comics, or that a ranking invites snobbery or valorizes a type of book learning or college reading, or that certain popular types have great subtlety. If discussions of this type are stimulated, and examples are suggested or rearranged, the enterprise of this ranking will only be the stronger for it. At the end of these rankings I shall return with practical help in using them.

Medical Uses of This Ranking. A more specific use to which this book is devoted is to aid us doctors in medically evaluating our patients with all types of psychiatric and neurological conditions. It is not a substitute for criterion-based psychiatric diagnosis, nor neurological and neuropsychiatric diagnosis employing anatomical imaging and physiological recordings. But an evaluation of a patient's sense of humor may give us a more emotionally and socially relevant measure of the living experience of the patient's reality and its impairment. Whereas our physical and mental status exams are tolerated if not understood, and sometimes experienced as off-putting or even threatening, I have found asking about what patients find funny is welcomed. Since this pertains to how their loved ones relate to them, families like it too. Asking about sense of humor can be upbeat and cheering at a difficult and frightening time for both patient and family, and thus therapeutic. As Norman Cousins described (1979) and *Reader's Digest* reminds us with its monthly feature, "Laughter [Is] the Best Medicine." It's also good practice.

Sensitivities and Triggers

Times are changing. In recent years the sensitivities of people in diverse and intersecting identity groups have led to social and legal prohibition of speech and other expression. The Christmas song, *Rudolph the Red Nosed Reindeer* (by Johnny Marks, 1949) is viewed as including bullying and *Baby, It's Cold Outside* (by Frank Loesser, 1944) viewed as suggesting sexual violation, as no not meaning no. Classic books are banned that appear to demean certain groups or trigger wounded feelings, especially on campuses. Title IX, once devoted to ensuring equal access to sports at colleges and other institutions that receive Federal money, is now applied to language and behavior that is felt to harm or demean. The criterion of violation is neither the intent nor the content but the subjective hurt of the victim(s). This rule has repeatedly been stressed and illustrated at Title IX training sessions at the Columbia Medical Campus and elsewhere.

There is usually a butt of a joke. Humor by its very nature, especially in standup routines, has often pushed the limits of acceptability to play upon our attitudes and taboos, both outrageously and beneficially. But now it is subjected to critiques based on awareness of harms felt by its targets.

The problem with humor, all the more in these sensitive times, is that by its very nature it usually has targets. Henri Bergson (1900, 1924) defined a basis for humor in deviance from social expectations and thought humor made us better persons. The socially deviating person is the target laughed at. This begs the question of whose social norms are held up as standard, and how broadly inclusive they are. Humor seldom has no one as its butt. The novelist Joyce Carol Oates (2008) said of Steve Martin, "what is most impressive about Steve is that, greatly gifted as he is in comedy, his comic
vision is essentially unifying--radiantly goofy, never injurious to anyone. It has become a rare comedy that doesn't trade upon marginalizing & insulting others." Dave Barry (Barry 2019) is a thankfully perennial supplier of laugh-out-loud but acceptable humor.

While such humor is possible, and Jim Gaffigan is yet another family-friendly practitioner who does segments on *CBS Sunday Morning*, one measure of the times is the struggle in this climate of the 115-year old Friars Club in New York, home to the royalty of American comedy and Milton Berle-member jokes

(Abrams 2019).

This ranking of humor will not be based upon acceptability, or violation versus innocuous fun. But the criterion of sensitivity violation remains relevant nonetheless, because of the priority given to empathy as a cognitive and neurological capability. Cruelty or crudity in humor as a result of a lack of empathy ranks lower and may reflect deterioration of the mental state. Or, it must be said, in some people there is brutishness from the get-go.

A caveat here: while ignorance of the law is usually no excuse, unintended sensitivity violations may be committed, especially by those far from language policing and campuses, such as older persons or those recently arrived in our American society. So we might bear in mind an accessory criterion of **awareness** or **wokefulness**, the absence of which, **cluelessness,** might more indicate being out of touch with contemporary manners than impairment or conscious cruelty. Psychiatric mental status exams have always asked such things as the names of Presidents or events in the news. We might also take note of patients' awareness of speech mores in the light of their social context. This can require tact.

Social significance. The capacity to appreciate humor is socially necessary, and underappreciated as a basis for our human connection. It is a marker of social bonding, of affirmation, of inclusion and exclusion, of belonging. As will be discussed, it is a highly socially relevant indicator of cognitive and neurological integrity. Although more complex than the usual abstract mental tests we use, such as the Mini-Mental State Exam MMSE) or the Montreal Cognitive Assessment (MoCA), the very social contingency of the sense
of humor makes it more relevant to a person's all-important social adaptation.

The social relevance of other tests of neurological status might also be more appreciated. For example, the practical Fahn pull test for postural instability (see Appendix) has much emotional and social relevance, in addition to its diagnostic use in evaluating physical balance in neurological conditions. Steadiness on one's feet is crucial to the feeling of security in older and neurologically impaired persons, and psychological experiments have demonstrated a presumed impact on relationships with significant others (see Appendix, below; Forest AL, Kille DR et al, 2015; Munhoz RP et al., 2004, and Forrest DV, 2007).

Obstacles to use in medical interviewing.

Cultural specificity of much humor can be a hurdle. A sensitive interviewer who speaks the patient's language can ask the patient to explain their examples, which can then be ranked. It is similar to the way we psychiatrists ask interviewees to interpret proverbs to evaluate abstracting ability. We may have to adapt sayings to the person's culture, or even ask them to suggest one. For example, Hispanic patients may find "Rolling stones gather no moss" or "People who live in glass houses shouldn't throw stones" very odd, but often cotton to "The shrimp that falls asleep gets carried away by the stream." They give such socially relevant abstract answers as "One should think for oneself and not be swept along by the mob," or "One should keep alert to opportunities to stand out from the crowd and move up." Asking patients to elaborate helps to evaluate abilities for humor and abstracting.

Education level and literacy are other factors to be taken into account. But the rank of humor that a person appreciates need not correspond to their educational level. An ingenious evaluator can improvise examples analogous to the rather literary ones I supply below, that are drawn instead from the person's world, such as real life situations, current events and subtle human interest stories they find funny or
ironic. These can be equally demanding and subtle.

Universality of ranking would derive then not from the examples, which may be culture-bound, or somehow idiosyncratic, but from the commonality in all of us of the cognitive processes and their neurological correlates.

To begin, an open invitation to provide a person's own

examples provides a jumping-off place. In trying examples from the levels below or analogous substitutes, it is best to start with easier ones. Keeping the person's educational level in mind, choose examples that are not challenging or arcane or snobbish. We create a spirit of acceptance, don't flunk people.

Ask the patient what they find funny on TV or the newspaper. Perhaps they will not be able to explain why something is funny, as this could be on another level of (metacognitive) thinking about thinking. Be prepared to learn; the patient may see a subtlety the interviewer missed. As the evaluation proceeds, more challenging stimuli can be tried.

Evaluating sense of humor--A caution

"Plop, plop, fizz, fizz, oh what a relief it is!" --Alka Seltzer jingle, by Thomas W. Dawes, wordmarked April 15, 1976.

Before we descend to rank lower and lower echelons of humor in others and ourselves, I caution against worry or headaches if *you* laugh at examples at the lower levels.

The level of the humor has little to do with how funny it is in a laugh-out-loud sense. I'll confess to finding the slapstick pacing of the 6 *Sharknado* films (Syfy films, 2013-18) funny, but comfort myself that I also appreciate humor at higher levels. Thus in evaluating a person's sense of humor, the adages apply that:

Absence of evidence is not evidence of absence (of capacity at that level); and

Presence of evidence is evidence of presence.

That is, finding the highest level of humor understood and appreciated is a useful sign of intactness of the function of the corresponding brain regions.

And laughing at lower forms of humor does not mean one's capacity is low, unless one cannot also laugh at higher humor. Or at least get the idea and smile to oneself.

A caveat and invitation

Disagreements may arise about the inclusion, omission and placement of examples at the levels. I invite suggestions for reclassification and rearrangement, and especially improvisation of other examples. My intent was to characterize levels for neuropsychiatric purposes, not to reign as a literary critic. It's the principles that are key.

The Rankings:
Rating of 4: Social Awareness
Figure: The highest and most demanding level of humor

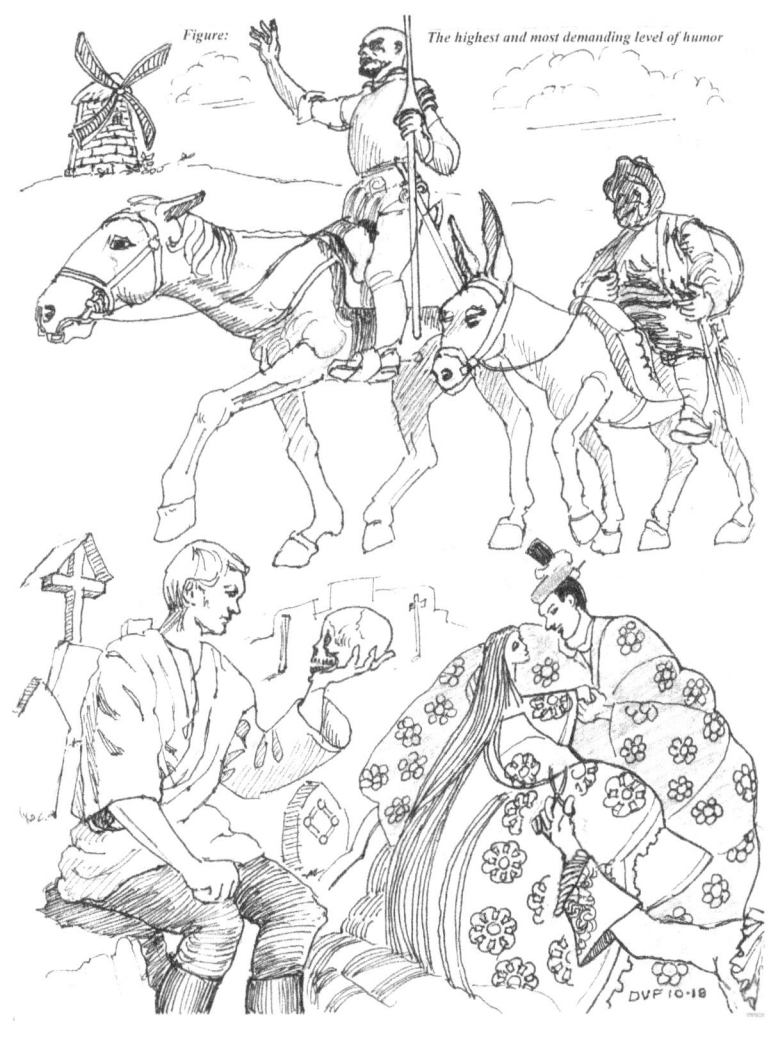

Figure: The highest and most demanding level of humor

Clockwise from bottom left: Hamlet *in the graveyard,* Don Quixote, The Tale of Genji *and Pope's* The Rape of the Lock. *A footnote to this illustration for me is the striking resemblance of Don Quixote, in the Madrid statue, from which I made the drawing, to Lenin, who was getting major traction when the statue was commissioned in 1915 by Spain's King Alfonso XIII to commemorate the 300th anniversary of the publication of Part II of the Quixote. King Alfonso, a Christian Monarchist, was no friend of communism, as his long political history proved. so it is ironic to see the most quixotic man in literature portrayed in the lineaments of Lenin. As well as photos, many statues of Lenin exist, and most of them, although mounted on horseback, besides having a similar face and head as the Don's, mimic the noble attitude of this pose, with his flexed left arm, and outstretched right arm. Lenin's open right hand differs in being a bit supinated as if to say "Lo and behold" while the Don's open right hand suggests a reaching and yearning gesture. Of course, the Lenin statues came later than the Don's, and the Spanish rightly revere Cervantes and his lofty fool above all others in literature. Their king likely would not have wished the Don to resemble anyone else, including Lenin, who later, according to the article by Albert Resis in The Encyclopedia Britannica, "must for good or ill be regarded as the century's most significant political leader." And if Communism is quixotic, it has surely been no joke.*

High/Highbrow Humor is humor that encapsulates unusually deep insights about people and the world, and appeals to those who are the most cultivated, tasteful and erudite. Empathy is ideally required and the quality of mercy is not constrained. Humor that approaches universal truth or applicability rather than narrow self-reflection warrants this rating. In Shakespeare's *Hamlet* (ca. 1600), Hamlet is in a graveyard holding and contemplating a skull he has just learned is that of

Yorick, his erstwhile court jester, and reminiscing about having kissed his lips. The conflation of this graveyard humor turns our stomach, but where in literature is our universal human mortality better brought home?

"Alas, poor Yorick! I knew him, Horatio; a fellow of infinite jest, of most excellent fancy; he hath borne me on his back a thousand times, and now, how abhorred in my imagination it is! My gorge rises at it. Here hung those lips I have kissed I know not how oft. Where be your jokes now? Your gambols? Your songs? Your flashes of merriment that were wont to set the table in a roar? Not one to mock your own grinning? Quite chapfallen." (William Shakespeare, *Hamlet, A Prince of Denmark* Act V, Scene i).

And how better to begin our foray into humor! Hamlet's musing about our mortality is the more excruciating because it's the skull of the loved jester he imagines having kissed, and because he chains outrageous *double entendre* ironies in mock jibes--Yorick's skull, like all skulls, is grinning, and Hamlet taunts Yorick for not mocking his own bony grin. Most precisely devastating is Shakespeare's choice of the word *chapfallen* (orig. chopfallen), which metonymically conveys dejection by a person's lower jaw hanging loosely--as we realize how loosely, with rotted muscles, a skull's jaw hangs.

This level of humor appeals most to educated people of generous spirit who are mentally and emotionally intact. It is not enough that they get the jokes. An empathetic tear must come to the eye, in coming, with Hamlet, literally face to face with death and loss. The humor becomes unbearingly poignant, and illustrates the emotional complexity of humor at the highest level.

A few more examples: "You don't realize you're intelligent until it gets you into trouble" ("James Baldwin: Reflections of a Maverick," Interview with Julian Lester *New York Times*, 27 May 1984); "If you think healthcare is expensive now, wait until...it's free," and "Term limits aren't enough: we need jail," (P.J O'Rourke, *The Liberty Manifesto,* Cato Institute speech,

May 6, 1993); and Ben Franklin's remarks on the pleasures of older women.

Humor about status reversals, often British, where there is great awareness of received societal pecking order, is found in P. G. Wodehouse, whose Reginald Jeeves is the highly competent valet of wealthy and idle Londoner Bertie Wooster (*Right Ho, Jeeves*, 1934). This is humor spelled humour.

Ian Fleming's James Bond is a working class agent who one-ups his aristocratic superiors M and Q with his knowledge of wines and history, and wins fortunes with ease on the gambling floor. Similarly, in Bong Joon-Ho's 2019 darkly comic *Palm d'Or*-winning masterpiece *Parasite,* a gullible upper-class family is snookered by a scheming envious underclass clan. There is a hint of at least erotic envy in the other direction. Highest level ethnic humor requires acute social sensibilities (see discussion of ethnic humor under Put Downs, below). Jordan Peele's 2017 film *Get Out*, which won Best Original Screenplay, depicts excruciating racial micro-aggressions before its horror bloodbath.

Don Quixote by Miguel de Cervantes (Part 1, 1605; Part 2, 1615) was the first modern novel. Harold Bloom, who was our pre-eminent literary critic, said of Cervantes that only Shakespeare comes close to his genius. *Don Quixote* couples humorous social awareness with idealism and pathos. Considered a funny book from the 17th Century, it is a picaresque novel in which a man of low social class pursues a "quixotic" quest in a fraudulent chivalric society. By 1813 Sismondi saw it as not just sad but *"le livre plus triste qui ait jamais été écrit" (Bardon, 1931).* Great humor is emotionally complex, and *Don Quixote* is both absurd humor and the tragedy of human aspiration and ambition. We can be surer of the greatness of a work when its title or author becomes part of the language. *Quixotic* describes that which is exceedingly unrealistic, idealistic, visionary, utopian, starry-eyed or impractical.

Similarly, Franz Kafka's (1883-1924) stories were also deemed hilarious when they were written. *Kafkaesque,* first used in 1939, is defined by Merriam-Webster as "anxiety, alienation and powerlessness of the individual in the 20th century. Kafka's work is characterized by nightmarish settings in which characters are crushed by nonsensical blind authority. Thus, the word *Kafkaesque* is often applied to bizarre and impersonal administrative situations where the individual feels powerless to understand or control what is happening." Metaphorically encapsulating this in stories like "The Trial" (1914) Metamorphosis" (1915) and "The Castle" (1922), Kafka made the bumbling bureaucracy of the crumbling Austro-Hungarian Empire darkly humorous then..

The Tale of Genji, written by Lady Murasaki Shikibu, a Japanese noblewoman of Chinese sensibility circa 1000 in the Heian Period, was the world's first novel and perhaps the best. It describes the adventures of Genji, a shining figure, son of the Emperor and a concubine who dies. Genji has many affairs from broadly comical to tragic. His father chooses a new Empress who reminds him of Genji's mother, and Genji has an affair and a son with her--surely as Oedipal a tale as one might wish--and the son rises in the Court as illegitimate Genji could not. The language is marked by word play and simultaneous complex emotions (contrasting with our usual Western sequential emotions), and the ending is ambiguous.

Requires (for appreciation of this level of humor): intact empathic emotional response of the limbic system; higher cortical function, especially constructional ability (in a far larger sense than parietal lobe figure copying) and integration of affects with cognition; intactness of the social perception circuit, which includes the fusiform gyrus and superior temporal sulcus (Björnsdotter, et al., 2016); appreciation of situational irony and verbal metaphor; and frontal lobe working memory. The primacy of empathy requires having had good enough rearing patterns and socialization for this capacity to have been laid down and well developed.

High Comedy, George Meredith's term in his *The Idea of Comedy* (1877), is an elegant and urbane comedy of manners in which the appeal is to the intellect primarily with a combination of grace and wit. Shakespeare's *Much Ado About Nothing*, Molière's *Tartuffe*, Austen's *Pride and Prejudice*, Mann's *The Magic Mountain* (Cudden, p. 308) qualify. Also Jacques Tati in *Mr. Hulot's Holiday (Les Vacances de Monsieur Hulot)*, a 1953 film in which Roger Ebert (November 10, 1996) found "an amused affection for human nature." *The Rape of the Lock* (1712-1714), a humorous narrative poem by Alexander Pope, describes a time of prissy baroque sensibility when great importance, tragedy and offense were laid to trivial matters of speech and slight offenses of comportment, perhaps not entirely distinguished from our own time. No doubt a male swine of an undergraduate today would be expelled or worse for doing what the Baron did, snipping a lock of Belinda's hair in fetishistic admiration. *The Rape of the Lock* is written in a mock-heroic style with classical references, such as treating the snipped hair with great importance, as if it were Helen of Troy. Termed by some **High Burlesque**, the poem satirized the pretentiousness of society, a universally applicable theme. Even its title risks trigger warnings today.

Requires: Knowledge of the manners of the society portrayed and the nuances of their violation. Henri Bergson in his *Laughter (Le Rire)* (1900), thought all humor was deviation from social norms. Cf. **Low Comedy.**

Irony - the meaning is contrary to the words, and not always funny. Examples: *Don Quixote, Tom Jones, Moll Flanders.* Prominent with the growth of satire in late 17th and early 18th Century; a high degree of sophistication.

Situational irony occurs in Iago's speech to Othello about himself sleeping next to Cassio. The deceptive Iago stokes Othello's jealousy by describing Cassio taking his hand and throwing his leg over him as though he were Othello's wife Desdemona--during which supposed drawn-out encounter, Iago keeps letting it happen without waking Cassio and telling him he is mistaken (*Othello* Act 3, Scene 3).

There is often "a discrepancy between words and meaning, actions and results, appearance and reality" (J.A. Cuddon, pp. 335-340). One of the loveliest and most touching examples of irony is Shakespeare's Sonnet 130: "My mistress' eyes are nothing like the sun;/ Coral is far more red than her lips' red;/ If snow be white, why then her breasts are dun;/ If hairs be wires, black wires grow on her head." It parodies the extravagant (racial) praise of other Elizabethan love lyrics but concludes, "And yet, by heaven, I think my love as fair/ As any she belied with false compare." Irony can be so subtle it can tax the patience and focus of the reader. Henry James's story, The Aspern Papers "investigates" the dilemmas that bring writers and readers together--and keep them apart" (James, 1983) in all the lovely prolixity of his sentences.

Sarcasm, overused by adolescents who have just learned it, betrays opposite meaning by tone of voice.

Requires: a sense of orientation to language and situations beyond literality. Contemplation of more than one level of meaning in comparison and contrast. Working memory in the dorsolateral prefrontal cortex must contain the elements and their contexts of expectation to be contrasted, and salience detection in the anterior cingulate gyrus must weigh how one element undermines, vitiates, defeats, or renders the other absurd.

Empathic overextension - this is a special category that could have been invented for Gary Larson. His cartoons are especially favored by scientists, although enjoyed widely. An extended analysis is given in the Appendix, but suffice to say he imagines in his cartoons the sensibilities and situations of both human and non-human consciousness, such as animals and aliens. Thus in one cartoon a group of dog scientists are studying the doorknob principle. His depiction of Scientist Hell shows a bearded white-coated new arrival, escorted by the devil, entering a room on the glass door of which is written "Psychics, Astrologists & Mediums Eternal Discussion Group". While those of a nerdy scientific bent may lack empathy, and even be on the autistic spectrum, in which a theory of others' minds is lacking, Larson's astonishing forays into the land of the *pathetic fallacy* reaches them. *The New Yorker* cartoons of dogs and cats by George Booth, who had a retrospective at The Society of Illustrators in New York in 2018, also empathically conveys so much about dogs by drawing one just sitting with its back to us, facing the front door, waiting where its master left and will return.

Requires: empathic imagination, perhaps the *negative capability* described by the Romantic era poet John Keats in 1817 (see Appendix re Larson), and *mind-mindfulness,* a less clinical way of saying Theory of Mind. This is the ability to sense and construct a reasonable idea of what another person (or creature) would be thinking, rather than assuming that they think and know what one thinks and knows oneself.

Satire (Cuddon, pp. 598-603) was defined by Samuel Johnson's dictionary as a poem "in which wickedness or folly is censured," and Dryden thought its true end was "the amendment of vices." It attempts (Cudden, p. 599) "to correct, censure and ridicule the follies and vices of society and thus to bring contempt and derision upon aberrations from a desirable and civilized norm." Aristophanes (448-380 BCE) wrote immortal satirical comedies, such as *The Frogs* (405 BCE) in which Dionysus travels to Hades to bring back Euripides, but decides instead, with a chorus of frogs, on the instructive values of the former classical glories of Aeschylus. In *Lysistrata* (411 BCE), women withhold sex to end the war between Athens and Sparta. In *Clouds* (423 BCE), the birds are convinced to give up their freedom, a satire of Athenian interventional politics. Jonathan Swift (1667-1745), Alexander Pope (1688-1744), Voltaire (1694-1778), Samuel Butler (*Erewhon,* 1872), and George Orwell (*Animal Farm,* 1945), are among the greatest satirists. Satire waxes and wanes through history; it declined after the ancients and in the 20th Century because of violence and instability. Swift's *A Modest Proposal* (1729) would end hunger in Ireland by eating the babies. Charlie Chaplin's *The Great Dictator* (1940) satirized Hitler.

Humorous social observation - One of the funniest and most iconoclastic works, trenchant because its commentaries and cartoons targeted us so well, was Paul Fussell's (1983) *Class: A Guide Through the American Status System..* From his British origins, Fussell brought his class consciousness with nary a doubt about his stereotypes, but the book was important and very popular because it challenged our American wishful myth of classless social equality. Our myth, like most myths, is maintained with great effort. However much mischief it may cause, we favor explaining all social status inequality by unfairness or victimization. But our myth is sacred to us, and is central to our national nobility and exceptionalism, however unrealized and unrealistic it might be. Fussell at his most British asserts that class is inevitable from birth and upbringing, and does not change however much money one gains or loses. He unceremoniously divides [white] Americans into Uppers, Middles and Lowers, whom he calls "Proles." There are subdivisions like the Top Out of Sight and the Bottom Out of Sight (incarcerated), both of whose offspring are reared by the same people. The Proles' literature of supermarket tabloids is the most interesting, and the Uppers' the most boring, limited to the social and yacht registries. The Middle Class living room in 1983 could be evaluated by the presence of Tutankhamen effigies, and the Proles' clothing was legible, inscribed with logos. *Class* is chock full of audacious *aperçus,* such as that one's social class is inverse to the diameter of the ball one plays with. The offensiveness of all this snobbery to American ears may be mitigated by realizing how much indeed we try to amplify our own social status, instead of feeling anchored in our place the way Europeans do. Bully for us, Brit!.

Other examples of social critique at this level are Tom Wolfe's (1975) *The Painted Word,* about the scam of contemporary art replacing skill with works needing jargon verbiage, and Lisa Birnbach's (1980) *The Preppy Handbook*, ridiculing the valorization of private school. A commentary-memoir, notable mainly because the author, Wednesday Martin, Ph.D. is an anthropologist and primatologist, is *The Primates of Park Avenue: Adventures Inside the Secret Sisterhood of Manhattan Moms* (2015), in which Lulemon-clad matrons intimidate one another by possessing the ultimate totem, a Hermes Birkin handbag. Preppy became an imitated style.

Requires: knowledge of the target of the satire and realization that the author does not always literally mean what is said. Extensive social awareness is needed, and the ability to read symbols and metaphors. Emotional
control may be needed to observe oneself unoffended.

Repartee-- quick and witty comments or replies (from the fencing term for answering a sword thrust), also termed banter, badinage, ripostes, quips, raillery, persiflage, comeback, rejoinder. Examples: Bernard Shaw pushed his way past a fat man on a narrow staircase. "Pig!" said the fat man angrily. Shaw tipped his hat and said, "Shaw, Good afternoon." (Cuddon, p. 564). This is a literal example, that is, on a staircase, of what Diderot called "staircase wit." Mohammed Ali, being refused to be served a hamburger and told, "We don't serve negroes," replied "That's OK, I don't eat 'em" (https://www.reddit.com). An instant comeback.

Requires: appreciation of rapid wit, *le mot juste* (Flaubert). Requires rapid cerebral working memory processing, intact dopaminergic system, substantia nigra.

Rating of 3-4: Situational Wit, Barbed Wit, Smaller Social Targets

Deadpan/Dry--witty humor delivered without smirking affect, often in an offhanded or reserved manner, as in a British drawing room comedy. Examples are James Bond's style of wisecrack after dispatching an adversary and Jack Benny, in his classic si-Sy-Sue dialog with Mel Blanc in a stereotypical Hispanic accent. Lovable grifter Barbara Stanwyck in Preston Sturges' 1941 comedy *All About Eve,* says of her mark and lover Henry Fonda's character, "I need him like an axe needs a turkey." In 1970 the Australian writer Irina Dunn coined the phrase, "A woman needs a man like a fish needs a bicycle," which was popularized by Gloria Steinem and adopted by feminists. "Monty Python's John Cleese sometimes does deadpan, but mostly maintains comic dignity during uncontrollable situations. His character is overwhelmed and excitable in the madcap *Fawlty Towers.* Bob Newhart's trademark deadpan delivery in his role as Dr. Robert Hartley, a psychologist on the 1970's sitcom *The Bob Newhart Show,* was reprised in his appearances since 2013 on *The Big Bang Theory* as Professor Proton, a fictional TV 'Mr. Science.' Also deadpan was Jack Webb's *Dragnet* (1951-1970) police Sergeant Friday who asked for "just the facts ma'am." Jim Jarmusch's 2019 zombie comedy ("zom-com") film, *The Dead Don't Die* stars Bill Murray and Adam Driver as deadpan cops and Tilda Swinton as a laconic Scottish sword-wielding undertaker. Some of the zombies show more expression.

Requires: Being born British or just reserved probably helps, or having a sense (for the British) of improperly excessive emotions, such as (to the British) the expressiveness of other ethnicities. Intact affect perception is required to see the humor in its incongruous absence.

Droll--Honore de Balzac's *Droll Stories (La Comedie Humaine,* 1874, banned for obscenity in Ireland and Australia in 1901, and Canada in 1914), are ribald and Rabelaisian tales concerned with such themes as cuckoldry, and intestinal gas intentionally brought about postprandially by a mischievous host who blocked access to toilets by his house guests, and then enjoyed their discomfort.

Epigrammatic--humor expressed in witty economy and concision, as in Ogden Nash's "Candy is dandy, but liquor is quicker" (from his 1931 "Reflections on Ice Breaking," in Nash, 1995, p. 632, and perhaps no longer politically correct). Geary (2018), in a book about wit of various kinds, describes wordy Polonius's ironic "Brevity is the soul of wit" in Hamlet as the most famous observation about wit, and adds Dorothy Parker's "brevity is the soul of lingerie" as an irreverent gloss. At the 2012 Correspondents' dinner, Barack Obama said, "I was, of course, born in Hawaii (wink)," referring to his birther controversy and compressing the concision into a facial gesture. Swarner (1996, p. 24) compiled Yiddish epigrammatic wisdom (*Yiddishe chochma*), some of which are funny as well as ironic, for example, "If you have money, you are wise and good-looking and can sing well too" (*Az me hot gelt, iz men klug un shain un men ken gut singen*). I once bought froyo from a Pakistani proprietor on two successive days and complained that he charged me a dollar more the second time. He replied, "It is a larger amount sir, you are wealthy, and a handsome man, too!" Cf: "He who marries a wealthy woman pays for it."

Plays on words-- John Dryden distinguished true wit, which can survive the test of translation, from false wit, which cannot, as it is based on the relationship between words rather than between ideas. Wordplay can vary from silly and barely meaningful *Witzelsucht* in frontal lobe syndromes or the juvenile snickering of Beavis and Butthead in the cartoon of the same name (which could be placed at level 1-2) to the brilliant, as in Shakespeare's *Romeo and Juliet* when the mortally wounded Mercutio says to Romeo (Act 3, Scene 1): "Marry, 'tis not so deep as a well, nor so wide as a church door, but 'tis enough, 'twill serve: ask for me tomorrow and you will find me a grave man." It would seem the simile of a well is a gross exaggeration until the playgoer of Shakespeare's time hears the next comparison to a church door, which was contemporary slang for the gothic outline of the external female genital, which in turn brings home the well as another off-color reference, by a dying young man as sexual as any, whose graveyard humor is then amplified by his grave man pun. Another example is the rap singer Busta Rhymes at the 2017 Grammy Awards referring to Donald Trump as Agent Orange. Whether or not one likes Mr. Trump (who is partial to veterans, including us sprayed with that defoliant), the combination of personal caricature (red face and yellow hair making orange) and the toxic chemical responsible for so much disease among us Vietnam veterans, is a marvelously compressed poetic trope. A *double entendre*, or wordplay on a pluripotent concept making a double meaning, is often a low form of humor, but in Shakespeare it is elevated to genius, because it informs and is subsumed by his contexts.

Requires: knowledge of the multiple meanings of words, metaphorical (abstraction) capacity, knowledge of the referents, e.g. Elizabethan slang or Vietnam history. Language processing areas of the brain must be intact, especially Wernicke's area in the dominant temporal lobe cortex.

Farce--a light, humorous, quickly paced play that involves ludicrous situations, surprise, exaggeration, action and dialogue, with more plot than character development, mirthful humor rather than wit, aimed to provoke roars of laughter rather than smiles, as in Shakespeare's *Comedy of Errors, Taming of the Shrew, Twelfth Night* and *Midsummer Night's Dream* (Shaw, p. 156, Cuddon, pp. 263-266). Armando Ianucci's cruelly funny 2018 film, *The Death of Stalin,* is described as a farce by Anthony Lane in the March 19, 2018 *New Yorker,* but it might be called a lampoon for its caricatures of Krushchev (played by Steve Buscemi), Malenkov (Jeffrey Tambor) and others. Russia, which banned the film, may have considered it a travesty, claiming it false and distorted.

Requires: Knowledge of history and politics in the Socialist Republic, and willingness to appreciate the dark humor in the murderous jockeying for political correctness as Khrushchev came to power in 1953. Much cortical assembly and association of stored knowledge is needed.

Parody--a spoof with an imitative use of words or style or attitude in such a way as to make ridiculous (Cudden, 483-485). Examples are *Mad Magazine, Saturday Night Live's* political caricatures, Jonathan Winters, and impressionists. Aristophanes' *Frogs*, in addition to its satirical regime correction is "a tartly affectionate parody of Greek tragedy" (Mendelsohn, 2016). *Bored of the Rings,* is a parody of J.R.R. Tolkien by Henry N. Beard and Douglas C. Kenney (Signet, for *The Harvard Lampoon,* 1969). Peter Schickele's parodic PDQ Bach's "undiscovered" works, e.g. *Iphegenia in Brooklyn, Royal Firewater Musick, Hindenberg Concerto, Oedipus Tex, Goldbrick Variations,*

Shepherd on the Rocks With a Twist, The Magic Fruit, Rosenkavalier and Guildenstern, Concerto for Horn and Hardart, "Unbegun" Symphony, Fanfare for the Common Cold, Canine Concerto "Wachet, Arf!" ("Sleeping Dogs Awake"), *Chaconne à Son Goût,* and *Famous Last Words of Christ,* exemplify parodic naming. "PDQ," slang for "pretty damn quick," parodies Papa Bach's many triple-initialed offspring, such as C.P.E.

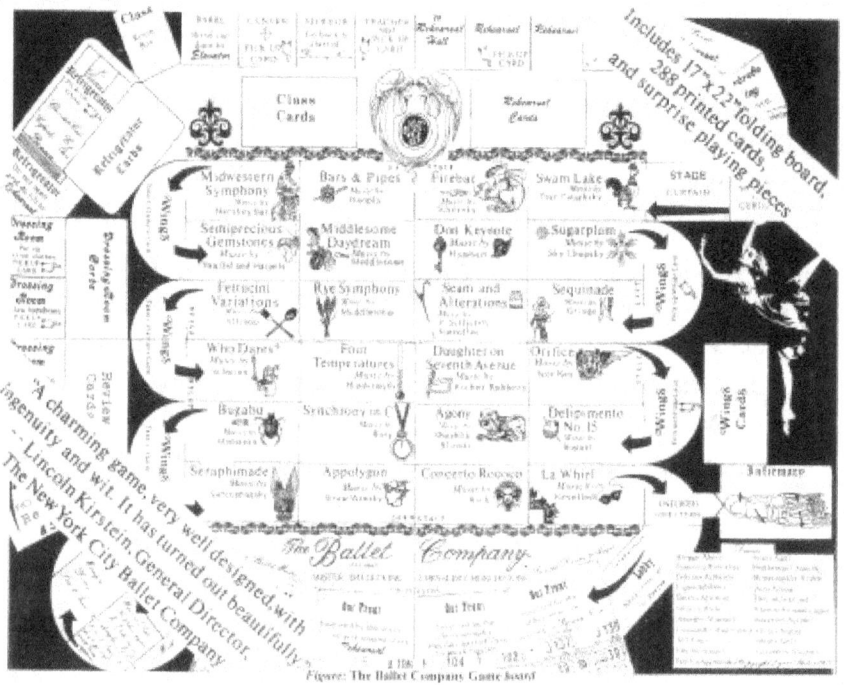

Figure: The Ballet Company game

Somewhat similar, but lovingly parodying the world of the classical ballet company in the form of a board game, is The Ballet Company Game (Lynne Stetson, 1976) which depicts the obstacles and triumphs in becoming a Balanchine ballerina, replete with word plays. Disclosure: Lynne Stetson, a former New York City Ballet dancer, is my wife and I collaborated in the design.

Figure: Key to the parodied names of Balanchine ballets in the previous Figure.

These correspond in position to the made-up names on the game board (the preceding Figure).

Frederick Crews parodies freudian analysis of literature in *The Pooh Perplex* (1963) and Peter Gay, who wrote *Freud: A Life for Our Time* (1988), also wrote a parody "lost" review of Freud's *The Interpretation of Dreams* that some have deemed a hoax. John Oliver wrote a gay spoof of a book by Vice President Mike Pence's daughter about the family bunny. She forgave him because the proceeds were donated to AIDS and LBTQ charities. Pence, who opposed gay marriage, didn't comment.

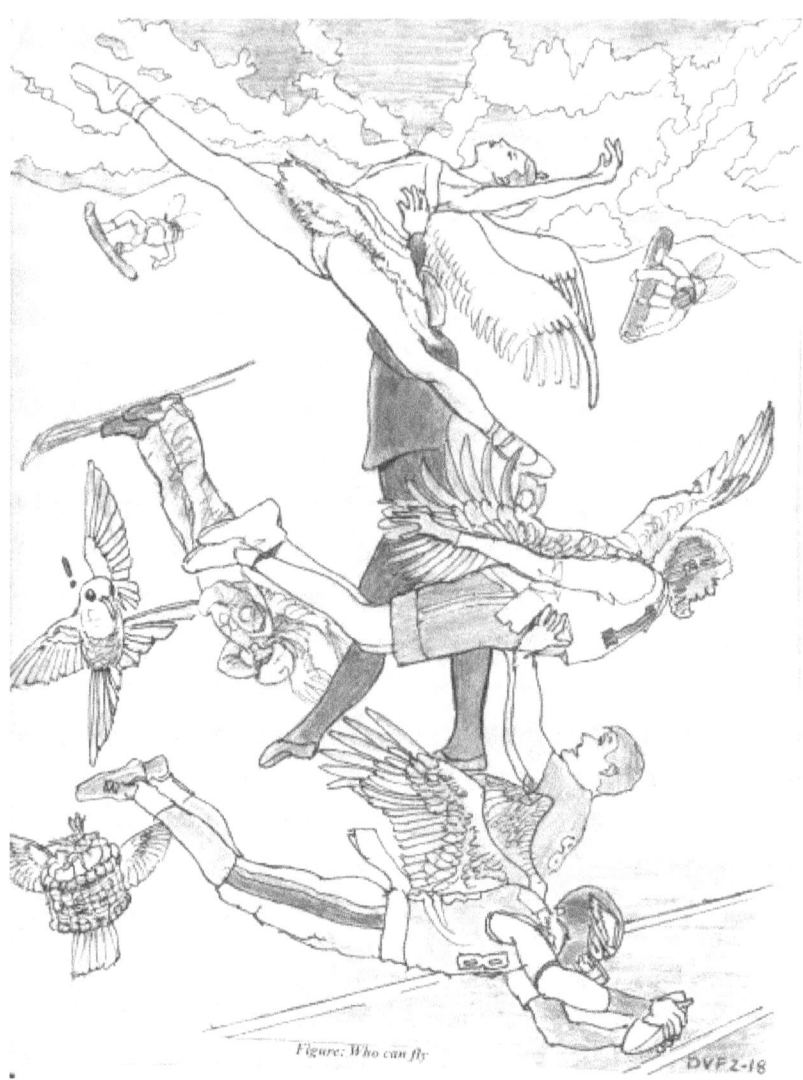

Figure: Who can fly

Figure: Who can fly

Parody is common in physical comedy. The best commercial of the 2018 Super Bowl was for the National Football League, and it featured legendary Giants quarterback Eli Manning and his astonishing wide receiver Odell Beckham Jr. spoofing Patrick Swayze's overhead lift of Jennifer Grey in the 1987 film Dirty Dancing *to the tune of "The Time of My Life." In the Figure, I gave Beckham wings, and also the other "flying" athletes: Zach Ertz in his diving 11-yard touchdown for the Philadelphia Eagles against the*

New England Patriots, to win the 2018 Super Bowl; Sara Mearns, lifted by Jared Angle in The New York City Ballet's Balanchine ballet, Symphony in C on January 20, 2018; Russian skier Liubov Nikitina in the women's aerial freestyle, and Red Gerard, who gold medaled in slope style, both at the 2018 Winter Olympics in South Korea. To amuse a French friend, I added wings to her favored recipe, vol-au-vent, or "flight in the wind," which consists of a very light puff pastry shell containing meat, fowl, game, or seafood in a savory sauce. This humorous assemblage yokes the heterogeneous together, as was favored by the 17th Century Metaphysical poets, and illustrates incongruity as a basic ingredient of humor.

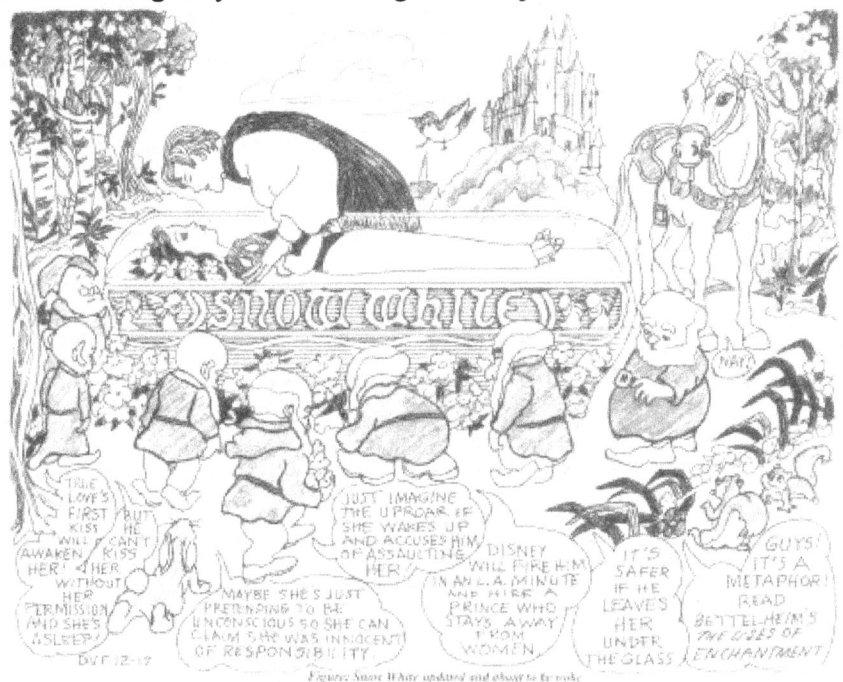

Figure: Snow White updated and about to be woke

A parody cartoon in the style of Disney depicts the moment the Prince bends over to kiss Snow White. The onlooking Seven Dwarves voice caution in today's climate of women's complaints about men. They say, "Love's first kiss will awaken her!" "But he can't kiss her without her permission and she's asleep!" "Maybe she's just pretending to be unconscious so she can claim she was innocent of *responsibility," "Just imagine the uproar if she wakes up and accuses him of assaulting her!" "Disney will fire him in an L.A. minute and hire a Prince who stays away from women," "It's safer if he leaves her under the glass." The last dwarf implores, "Guys! it's a metaphor! Read Bettelheim's* The Uses of Enchantment.*" This classical psychological study (Bettelheim, 1976) psychoanalyzed fairy tales as emotional instruction for children, signifying their journey of maturation, culminating in the awakening of genital sexual sexuality and mastery over the kingdom of the self (The cartoon was displayed in the Columbia University Irving Medical Center Art Exhibit, 2018-2019).*

As a Princeton undergraduate, I had the pleasure of writing a thesis (Forrest, unpublished ms., 1960) for the English Department about E. E. Cummings, and to have had the poet's help with it. In it I proposed that Cummings's poetry favored three emotional attitudes, appearing in his ever-shifting dramatic voices, of wonder, nausea and fun. The last two attitudes appeared in devastating irony, mock and sardonic addresses, and parody. Parodying political speeches, his "next to of course god america i" (Cummings, 1991, p. 367) has become for me an unforgettable translucent overlay upon almost all politicians' speeches, laden as they are with sanctimony, testimony, and platitudinous rant. In fragments segued together in a manner reminiscent of Schickele's musical everything-but-the-kitchen-sink, *Quodlibit,* Cummings's politician works in "land of the pilgrims," "my country 'tis," "these heroic happy dead/who rushed like lions to the roaring slaughter," and "the voice of liberty." The last line is, "He spoke. And drank rapidly a glass of water." Cummings' ear for cant was applied to all group thinking.

Another example of self-styled parody was Congressman Adam Schiff"s September 26, 2019 retelling of Donald Trump's phone call with Ukranian President Zelensky "partly in parody" in the form and tone of a mobster coercion.

Requires: Knowledge of musical, historical, political or literary referents. Comparative function as in humor generally.

Ability to stylize the parody close enough to the original to be convincing and humorous. Associational cortical areas. Requires an "ear" for speaking styles and tone.

Musicality can be a simple gift or a highly developed skill and has a parallel in **Physical empathy**, needed to appreciate physical comedy, discussed below under **Slapstick**.

Situational or sitcom--as in situation comedies, established characters find themselves compelled to deal with events constructed to test their character and interrelatedness. Stock characters in sitcoms typically "never learn" or develop, as they do in novels, plays and short stories, although they may somewhat in some of the better long series. Compare unchanging Jackie Gleason and Audrey Meadows in *The Honeymooners* (1955-1956) with *The Wonder Years* (1988-1993), which followed a cast of children over 5 years portrayed by Fred Savage, Josh Saviano and Danica McKellar. TV's *The Big Bang Theory* (2007-2019), about physics nerds and a waitress, has adapted some of its characters' never-learning traits for slight character development allowing for marriages between Bernadette and Howard, Penny and Leonard, and Amy and Sheldon; but the crime comedy series *Monk* (2002-2009) never permitted the titular obsessive-compulsive detective played by Tony Shaloub symptomatic relief. Producers of several hit sitcoms include Norman Lear in the 1970's (*All in the Family* with the Archie Bunker character, *Sanford and Son, The Jeffersons,* and *Maude*); and Chuck Lorre (*Two and a Half Men, Dharma and Greg, The Big Bang Theory, Young Sheldon,* and *The Kaminsky Method*).

Situational comedy is sensitive to the temper of the time. Neil Simon (1927-2018), deemed "The King of Stage Comedy" in *The Wall Street Journal* obituary feature of August 27, 2018 (Terry Teachout, p. A13), was America's most popular playwright for a quarter century, but his smash hits are now considered passé and not revivable, because of what *The New York Times* (in its obituary feature) described as "Big Laughs and Then a Shift in Culture" (Jesse Green, August 27, 2018, pp. C1,C4), and "a real story of male collapse that was relevant to the culture at the time."

In *Seinfeld,* a TV series which ran from 1989-1998, its narcissistic, morally adumbrated characters are so incorrigibly selfish that in the last episode, the producers leave them stuck together in a jail cell, bringing to mind Sartre's existentialist play *No Exit* (*Huis Clos,* 1944). *Seinfeld's* concluding episode is arguably morally retributive (Iannone, 2018) and, in its spoofing of contemporary pieties, politically incorrect.

Mad Men (2007-2015), the 1960s American period drama TV series (Lionsgate) produced by Matthew Wiener, featured Jon Hamm as Madison Avenue advertising man Don Draper. In the last episode of the last season, Don has fled McCann Erickson, the big ad firm that swallowed Don's firm, and he is working on a Coca-Cola ad. After a cross-country odyssey in which he does some good turns, he ends up in an Esalen-like California retreat overlooking the Pacific. He has assumed another soldier's identity, divorced two wives, seduced innumerable women, broken all his vows and scandalized his daughter. An everyman in a therapy group compares himself (and Don) to "refrigerator people" who sometimes open and the light goes on, suggesting his dark emptiness. Don uncharacteristically hugs him. In the penultimate scene, he is sitting in the lotus position on the top of a hill, presumably meditating, when he smiles slightly. The next scene is the world's most famous ad--the 1971 "Hilltop" Coca Cola ad (Bill Backer et al.), with people of all races singing, "I'd like to buy the world a home/And furnish it with love/Grow apple trees and honey bees/And snow-white turtledoves/I'd like to teach the world to sing/In perfect harmony/I'd like to buy the world a coke/And keep it company. It's the real thing/What the world wants today/ It's the real thing." Interpretations of this ending vary, but is there a new, realer Don? The producer and actor agreed that Don has discovered himself at last, but the real Don Draper is the advertising man who thinks up the commercial in a meditation haven. This bittersweet comic irony, which has been set up throughout the series, makes this perhaps the best ending of a situational series. Fish got to swim, ad men got to sell, and I couldn't stop smiling.

Insurance TV ads - Perhaps acknowledging that insurance is boring and hard to get people to think about, ads by insurance companies are among the funniest on television. Geico's may be the funniest, as they have moved beyond their gekko lizard spokescreature to scenarios of exaggeration and incongruity. (Disclosure: as a former military officer, I am insured by USAA and have no connection with Geico).

In one Geico ad, a secret agent runs around a rooftop eluding and fighting off multiple enemies, as a helicopter loudly approaches, He takes out his phone, and calling the chopper shouts. "Where are you?" while kicking away another attacker. Then we see his mom on the phone in her living room, calmly reporting "Well, there are squirrels in the attic again." "Mom?" he says. She drones on, "And your father won't call the exterminator." "What?" he says, "can I call you back?" The announcer says, "When you're a mom, you call at the worst possible moment. Its what you do. If you want to save 15% or more on your car insurance, you switch to Geico. It's what you do." The mom continues, "Where are you? It's very loud there. Are you taking a Zumba class?"

The contrast is triple: Secret agent, Mom, insurance.

In a Geico commercial that aired at the 2018 World Cup, a player who scored keeps absurdly sliding and sliding on his knees back and forth across the field while the announcer says, "as long as soccer players celebrate with a slide, you can count on Geico to keep on saving folks money on car insurance."

A girl at a science fair has opened up a wormhole through time, through which Marie Antoinette, futuristic creatures and a pterodactyl are emerging. One teacher is asking another if she can believe it, but when she asks if he is referring to the wormhole, he says, "No, I can't believe how easy it was to save hundreds of dollars on car insurance with Geico."

In a close up of a soap opera couple, she is crying and he says, solicitously, "Hey, what is it?" "She says, "I realize I love you but as long as you are with Jessica there can never be anything between us." He says, "Tess, there's no need to cry. I've got really great news." "You're leaving Jessica?" "No, I just saved a bundle on my car insurance by switching to Geico." As she walks off hurt, he adds, "I *saved*. I thought that *meant* something to you." An announcer says, "Fifteen minutes can save you 15% or more on your car insurance."

Requires: these parodic ads require a sense of the usual way things happen in the exaggerated situations shown, and a realization that in reality the emotionally imperative, attention-grabbing scenarios would not be incongruously compared and upstaged by the pedestrian concern about saving money on auto insurance. There is empathetic pleasure in seeing the secret agent being gentle and polite with his mom even in a death-defying situation. To be funny, the soap opera heel's disregard of his girlfriend's feelings requires the viewer to empathize with her and see his expectation of her being satisfied as absurd. The soccer ad demands knowledge of the conventional game behavior and the laws of physics that contradict frictionless, unabated sliding. It is perhaps a satiric comment on the emotionality and announcer's prolonged "go-o-o-o-o-o-o-o-al! go-o-o-o-o-o-o-o-al! when a goal occurs at last in soccer.

Farmers Insurance features astonishingly freakish happenings (like a moose attack) that result in property damage. The actor J.K. Simmons announces that "we covered it" and closes with the tag line, "We know a thing or two because we've seen a thing or two." This appeals to those who like disasters or enjoy *Schadenfreude* at accidents, much as in the TV show *America's Funniest Home Videos.* The gist is literally to threaten the viewer into insurance coverage, and would rank more simple and direct on the humor scale. The same with the destructive "Mr. Mayhem" Allstate commercials from 2010 played by Dean Winters ("Protect yourself from mayhem--like me!"), recently with Tina Fey;
and Dennis Haysbert's solemn "Are you in good hands?" commercials since 2004, also for Allstate.

Requires: Situational humor relies on knowledge of social norms and mores, tropes and clichés, but often not much memory of the characters' histories as they demonstrate who they are each episode. In period pieces knowledge of the issues of that day contributes. The humor in situational humor requires that the characters be believable, and a sense of character traits and their continuity is needed to laugh at them. A high degree of cortical and limbic brain intactness is necessary to detect irony and incongruity about the social situations portrayed in the insurance ads. Indeed, an ironically refined but ever-offended cave man in a multiple-episode Geico ad describes himself deservedly as "advertising royalty." I loved and was amused by this clever tragicomic character, so I sent its actor/comedian John Lehr a preprint of this book, He replied with a funny blurb I used on the cover.

High Ethnic Humor-Ethnic humor that is respectful and faithful to its subject, usually excused by being delivered by a member of the ethnic group being portrayed, must walk the line of avoiding deprecation. Some of the best African-American stand-up comics like Richard Pryor, Eddie Murphy or Chris Rock are edgy in this way. The risk of offense is always present. Whether the comedian gets away with it depends on the audience and setting, and may change over time. For example, Jackie Mason's humorous contrasts of Jews and Christians that delighted on a Broadway stage, offended at a political rally. One of the more adroit examples, both affectionate and trenchant, is Molly Katz's (1999, 2010) *Jewish as a Second Language*, which has a sprinkling of Yiddish definitions, but exhibits a keen ear for Jewish-American syntax and diction. Novak and Waldoks's *The Big Book of Jewish Humor* (1981) compiles a distinguished roster of Jewish humorists and mostly respectable humor, for example a *MAD Magazine* parody of *Fiddler on the Roof* entitled "Antenna on the Roof."

Universality is an attribute of highly ranked humor, or so I have proposed. Others might ask if there is even such a thing as Jewish, Irish, Cajun, or Down East humor. Jeremy Dauber's intended-to-be-definitive *Jewish Humor* (2017) considers Jewish humor to comprise: responses to antisemitic persecution, Jewish social satire, wit, crude humor, metaphysical irony, Jewish folk humor, and attempts to define Jewishness. Ethnic humor limited to in-group reference belongs lower in ranking than humor more universal to all humankind, even if it is about those oppressed or persecuted.

That being said, all humor has a setting and particularity. **Jewish Humor** is discussed further below. Lulu Wang's 2019 film, *The Farewell,* is about a family's typical Chinese efforts to conceal the grandmother's terminal illness from her. They stage a faux wedding so they can all visit her for the last time. The situational comedy depends, for its ironic humor, upon those cultural practices, well-explained in the film, and upon demonstrations by the unsinkable grandmother of *chi (qi)* energy. Only the love is universal.

Requires: High cultural/ethnographic competence, awareness of social norms and taboos, fresh observations, and empathic assessment of audiences. It also needs constant updating. Usually great linguistic skill is applied to echo ethnic nuances, and certainly to attempt dialects. Ability to play with stereotypes without creating slurs is key. Example:
Katz describes (p. 147) how her "5 Basic Types" of Jews pronounce the names of Jewish holidays: "Vanilla Jews: Don't mention them, but use the day off to play tennis; Regular Jews: Say them with no Hebrew Accent; New Jews: Pay for lessons to learn the correct accent; Very Jewish Jews: Say them with phlegm in all the right places; Even More Jewish Very Jewish Jews: Are too busy complaining to God to pronounce anything." Some audiences today would object to this humorous stereotyping, even by a member of the group.

High Gender Humor - Examples: Amy Schumer's or Roseanne Barr's standup on sexual themes. (A bigoted tweet about race cost Roseanne dearly in 2018).

Requires: constant updating with attention to changing gender norms and roles, and community/viewership tastes.

Barr lost her 2017 sitcom named for her over an atrociously racist put-down. Transsexual humor might be challenging for some audiences to understand, and gay humor that was based on internalized homophobia and self-ridicule may offend contemporary sensitivities. The world's oldest joke book was *Philogelos (The Laughter Lover)*, from 4th or 5th Century CE Greece, translated by John F. Quinn, 2001. It contained 265 jokes, none explicitly about homosexuals, but a category about "horny women" who, given choices, always choose sex. There are also **Put-Down** jokes (which see, below) in *Philogelos* about foolish intellectuals. For example, an intellectual bought a pair of pants (a virile barbarian fashion newly becoming popular at that time) and found they were too tight, so he plucked the hair around his legs (which was an effeminate practice, so possibly a put-down of effeminacy). There are also jokes about misogynistic men.

New Yorker and Similar Cartoons--These deserve a category of their own. Gordon Parker, M.D., Ph.D. (2016) wrote that they "seemingly carry a New York stamp, characters world-weary, droll, dryly astringent, or alternatively, overly materialistic, smug, or cynical." In a 2013 TED talk, *New Yorker* cartoon editor Robert Mankoff noted that the stereotypic *New Yorker* cartoon not only is playful but also presents a level of incongruity (e.g., polite syntax, rude message) and exudes a 'benign violation.'" The violation would be that of a cosmopolitan New York City sensibility. To my mind, the cartoons, while funny in a reserved way, are as restrained and tepid as that magazine's poetry. Diffee (2011) collected cartoons rejected by the *New Yorker*. They are more daringly funny. For example, one by Barbara Smaller (p. 108) shows a teenage daughter with her mother holding a box of baby mementos and saying "Here's a lock of your hair, your first tooth, and your placenta." Another by J.C. Duffy (p. 239) shows a man with one hand in a punch bowl and his other feeling the breast of a woman to whom he is saying, "I never know what to do with my hands at a party." In his introduction to Diffee's book, cartoon editor Mankoff wrote (p.

vii) of his "former friend" Diffee's rejection collection that it "is yet more proof that bad taste and humor are not strange bedfellows." Taboo and offensively low can be funny.

Women's *New Yorker* Cartoons

When some men say women lack a sense of humor, one might ask whether the humor at which they are supposed to laugh has women as its butt. And have women creators of humor been asked to contribute their body of work? Granted that in our primal function of reproducing our species, women cannot so lightly laugh off the risks of rolling in the hay, and it is their role in society to keep men from laughing too much.

To a list of liberated ladies of standup comedy, we might add an exhibit entitled "Funny Ladies of *The New Yorker* Then and Now" at The Society of Illustrators (July 24 to October 13, 2018), that dispels any doubt about women's humorous capabilities. I shall describe some examples to indicate the flavors of the exhibit. Ethel Plummer was *The New Yorker's* first woman cartoonist, and her work appeared in the inaugural issue in 1925, only 5 years after women won the vote. Publication of women's cartoons lagged until the 1960s and 1970s when William Shawn began to publish them. That being said, Helen E. Hokinson (1893-1949) published 1800 cartoons and 68 covers, and the "Hokinson women" she depicted with gentle humor are described in Wikipedia as "wealthy, plump and ditsy society women" and "the dowager denizens of women's clubs." In a cartoon at the exhibit, she shows a college-bound teen packing her trunk while her mother says, "I hope, dear, you won't come back from Vassar with a lot of <u>ideas</u>." Her captions were usually written by male editors. Mary Petty in the Society of Illustrators show depicts an entirely nude female model entering a studio, to whom the male artist says "Dear no, Miss Mulberry--just the head." Carolita Johnson depicts a girl about age 6 with a doll asking her mother who is dressing before a mirror, "Mommy, when will I blossom into a beautiful projection of male desire?" Marisa Acocella depicts two fashionable young women having a drink at a bar while one says "Been there, done him." Emma

Hunsinger has God overseeing his angels in heaven creating Adam from a blueprint with dotted circles where genitals and hair will be added, and saying, "Do you think 78% water is too juicy?" The Surreal McCoy (the artist's pseudonym) shows a hospital ward in which buffalo roam in a cartoon entitled "Therapy Buffalo."

To the extent that humor could be said to be women's humor, it would be thought less universal by half, but I think everyone would laugh at this exhibit with its often traditional women's themes of being seen, creating humans, and turning the tables on men. The same for men's humor and guy jokes.

Requires: As in appreciating *The New Yorker's* poetry, indulgence of New York-style urban manners, attitudes, refinement and standards, perception of nice differences, importance of minor shades of feelings and absurd juxtaposition. Topical themes and plays upon *au courant* passing language fads render some cartoons rapidly dated. One conceit is a trend toward cartoonists who can't draw well.

The Comics of the drawn-on-paper type could be inserted here at a high level, to reflect how they have evolved, funny-paper funny to edgy and disruptive social commentary. Some of the early classics like George Herriman's *Krazy Kat* (see Forrest, 2002) and Winsor McKay's *Dreams of the Rarebit Fiend* (see Forrest, 1987) combined brilliant commentary, language play and high illustrative art. Chute (2017) has chronicled the history and significance of the comics since Richard Outcault's *Yellow Kid* (1895-98 in Joseph Pulitzer's *New York* World) as art and literature, and noted how good they are at showing internal states, bodily taboos, urban life, historical catastrophes, whimsy, fantasy, non-realist adventure, and facial expression that text lacks. They have reached literary peaks, and are now often subtle, snarky, ironic and obscure, demanding knowledge of rapidly-changing styles and conventions, especially of those among young people. Comics now are free not to be so ha-ha funny, nor to need classification as humor in this categorization.

Rating of 3: Something Blue

Sexual jokes probably don't deserve to be classified at a lower level per se, but many people feel debased by them, especially if unwelcomed, and they are pathologically associated with intoxicated, manic, and demented brain states. the taking They can result from the taking dopamine agonists by dopamine-deficient Parkinson patients. In-group gay sex humor can contain self-deprecatory internalized homophobia. It is taboo-challenging to mention the unmentionable.

Blue Humor/Off Color Humor/Dirty Jokes--Chaucer's *The Miller's Tale* is as dirty as any humor, and its cuckolded carpenter is a severely-treated butt of it. Modern examples include stand-up comediennes Sarah Silverman and Amy Schumer, and Benny Hill's peeping bits. Hill was also notable for his verbal wit (see **Word Play**) and humorous accents that rival Sid Caesar's. At the beginning of my lifetime, pregnancy itself was considered off-color evidence of hanky panky, and to be hidden in confinement. Only recently comics Amy Schumer, Ali Wong and others have been appearing pregnant and joking about it (Harris 2019). For the ultimate in dirty humor, see **Appendix, The Aristocrats**, although the humor in that template is more about performing it and the ironic juxtapositions than the scatology per se.

Often the better off-color jokes are more implicit than explicit:

Lulabelle was the new hire fresh out of college at Chesebrough-Ponds, and the boys in marketing thought she should lead the focus group on their favorite product while they watched through the one-way mirror. Entering the room, she saw couples were as old as her parents. She opened the list of questions they gave her and her eyes widened. "How has Vaseline affected your love life?" she read, uncomfortably. After an awkward pause, one woman said, "Don't fret dear, I'll tell you. Vaseline has wonderfully improved our love life!" Lulabelle gasped as she read the next question: "Please be specific." Without a dropped beat, the lady said, "Well, we smear it on the doorknob so the kids can't get in."

So as not to dwell overly in the off-color valley at this point, I shall give the briefest of examples, told to me by a colleague never at a loss for humor:

At the end of time, the chicken and the egg spend the night together. The morning after, the chicken says to the egg, "Well, that settles it!" (If it hasn't come to mind, think of the eternal question).

Requires: Knowledge of what is appropriate sexual behavior, what is taboo and unmentionable; adjustments for the specific audience addressed. Comics walk the line on this and rely on an acute sense of gender differences and unspoken rules for social circles and mixed and diverse versus single-sex gatherings. For blue humor to be appreciated in its context when it is allowed, a joke's teller or listener needs a basic emotional impulse control, originating in the frontal lobes of the brain, to frame it.

Limericks--a form of rhyme-driven light verse, usually ribald, with a specified rhythm (anapestic) and meter (first, second and fifth lines trimeters, third and fourth dimeters). I was searching for one that did not employ "Nantucket" as a rhyme when I encountered Robert Elvove, M.D. (personal communication, May 3, 2016), who recited:

While Titian was mixing rose madder,
 His mistress went up on a ladder;
Her position to Titian
Suggested coition
So he went up the ladder and had 'er.

(An only slightly different version appears in Cuddon, p. 363). The amusement of a limerick is hardly its ribald sense, which in prose might be paraphrased, e.g., "A famous painter was mixing a hue when his mistress climbed a ladder, affording him a view of her lady parts, so he became aroused, joined her on the ladder, and they had sex." A person with aprosody or amusia would miss the rhythmic, rhyming effect. Aprosody means difficulty expressing or comprehending prosody, which is the melody of speech, including pitch, accent, and rhythm. Amusia is difficulty with music more specifically. 4% of us are tone deaf; others can't recall or reproduce a tune. And some, we'll see, lack a sense of humor.

Near rhymes are frequent as long as the meter-driven rhythm works:
> There was a young priest from Nigeria
> Who felt he was very inferior
> He did to a nun
> What shouldn't be done
> And now she's a Mother Superior.

That example illustrates that in addition to its prosody, a limerick is conventionally expected to be transgressive. Compare, and perhaps find too abstractly tepid:
> A dozen, a gross and a score
> Plus three times the square root of four
> Divided by seven
> Plus five times eleven
> Is nine squared and not a bit more.

Or, in Arabic numbers, a still less rollicking

$$\frac{12 + 144 + 20 + 3\sqrt{4}}{7} + (5 + 11) = 9 \times 9 + 0.$$

During World War II a limerick addressed the Nazi High Command, its limerick form as incomplete as its content:
> Hitler had only one ball
> Himmler had two but quite small
> And Goebbels had no balls at all.

Garrison Keillor, who became a target of Me Too accusations, supplied that one in the final show of his *Prairie Home Companion* on July 6, 2016, featuring imaginary Lake Wobegon, "where all the woman are strong, all the men are good-looking, and all the children are above average," a tag line that satirizes American (Midwestern) conceit and exceptionalism. He also supplied:
> There once was a man from Pocatello
> (whence many limerick people come)
> Whose urine was turning bright yellow

> Was it something I ate
> Or was it the date
> Last night with Kate? Hello!

More innocent, but similar to limericks, were the Burma-Shave sequential roadside signs. Burma-Shave, the shave cream, introduced them in 1925 and they amounted to 600 different ones in 7000 locations. These would be six 10" x 36" signs spaced 100 feet apart. The first five were a single line each of a rhyming jingle and the sixth was the cursive Burma-Shave logo. They lasted until 1963 when Burma-Shave was sold to Philip Morris, and the 1965 Highway Beautification Act marked their death knell. Rowsome (1965) collected all 600, some of which follow:

Past a schoolhouse/Keep it slow/Let the little/Shavers grow/Burma Shave

He played a sax/Had no B.O./But his whiskers/Scratched/So she let him go/Burma Shave

If Crusoe'd/ Kept his chin/More tidy/He might have found/A lady Friday/Burma Shave

You can drive/A mile a minute/But there is not/A future in it/Burma Shave

SLAP/THE JAP/WITH/IRON/SCRAP/Burma Shave

It's best for/One who hits/The bottle/To let another/Use the throttle/Burma Shave

The Wolf is shaved/So neat and trim/Red Riding Hood/Is chasing him/Burma Shave

Thus they range from public service announcements and WWII slogans to plugs for shaving and their cream.

Requires: intact prosodia (processing of language variations in speed, tone and emphasis) for limericks, and musia (processing of pitch for their jingle sound). Classed with aphasia, aprosody and amusia require left hemisphere function for timing and non-dominant hemisphere function for tone, pitch and emotional variation. The comedic pleasure is in the economy and the inevitability of the rhythm and the rhyme closure.

A variety of disorders can produce aprosody, including lesions and strokes affecting the right non-dominant temporal-parietal junction, childhood apraxia of speech, multiple sclerosis, and amyotrophic lateral sclerosis; and also such psychiatric disorders as schizophrenia, the autism spectrum, bipolar disorder and post-traumatic stress disorder.

Bedroom Farce/Sex Farce (the most common type of farce) is a type of light comedy centered on sexual pairings and swappings of characters as they move through improbable plots and slamming doors (Wikipedia). Examples are Arthur Schnitzler's play *Le Ronde* (1900), the BBC television series *Fawlty Towers* by John Cleeese and Connie Booth (1975 and 1979), Michael Frayn's *Noises Off* (1982), and the "Love Car Displacement" episode of *The Big Bang Theory* (Season 4, Episode 13, first aired 20 Jan 2011). Scottish author George Macdonald Fraser (1925-2008) wrote the *Flashman Papers,* a series of 12 books published from 1969 to 2005, in which the protagonist is a cowardly cad who improbably rises, in a series of historically-based adventures set between 1839 and 1894, to become a brigadier general, to influence history, and to bed 480 women by the 10th volume.

Requires: Memory of characters and a reasonably nuanced sense of their probable vs. improbable pairings.

Dirty Jokes--sexual innuendo, scatological, toilet humor, genital, phallic, urological humor. The notorious joke, "The Aristocrats" (see **Appendix**) is not a simple dirty joke because the intent is to contrast obscene behavior with the punch line label. Here's a simple dirty joke that takes a moment to get:

Farmer Brown was sleeping soundly after a hard day's farm work when Mrs. Brown woke him up. "Ezra, somebody's stealing our pumpkins, you better get up!" He got up wearily, pulled on his overalls, and got his shotgun. As he approached the pumpkin patch, he saw a tall stranger not stealing, but having his way with his prize pumpkin. "Stop or I'll shoot!" Farmer Brown ordered. The stranger paused, stood up, looked down at the pumpkin, and then at his watch. "Damn," he said, "It's after midnight!"

Requires: an intact "dirty mind," and a sense of what decency is being transgressed. Intactness of frontal lobe application of social standards is necessary for realization of the transgression. Impairment of frontal lobe function, or lack of inhibition as a result of intoxication or mania, could result in gross indecent humor, but the lack of a frame of reference will be evident. The above example requires familiarity with the Cinderella fairy tale, which began in China and is very international, if not universal (see Forrest, 1971).

Guy jokes (if humor can be gendered) have a self-conscious, usually boyish and brutish perspective:

An engineer down at Amalgamated Bra Corporation came up with a design that abolished jiggling once and for all, and prevented anything showing through on even the coldest days. But the genius didn't make it to the product launch. On the way, a bunch of guys beat the crap out of him.

Rating of 2-3: Assassinations

Placing humor that features cruelty, sadism or retribution lower in ranking may be justified to the extent that it lacks empathy. Callousness and cruelty can be acquired.

Dante Alighieri's *La Divina Commedia,* or **The Divine Comedy** (1308) must be considered in this ranking, not the least because its title contains the word comedy, which comes from the Greek for a merrymaking poet or singer, and means a poem or story with a happy ending. Classical revival in the 16th Century brought back the sense of the humorous and ridiculous known in antiquity. When my college classmates and I first read the *Commedia,* we loved best and dwelt most upon the first of its 3 books, *Inferno,* preferring it to the ever-brightening fireworks finale of *Paradiso,* or the Seven Deadly Sins of *Purgatorio,* with Dante's own groveling apologies for the wayward strayings of his own youth. No, *Inferno* encouraged our callow leanings toward the Rabelaisian, the Gargantuan, the gross, the cruel. In those days at Princeton we were unleavened by any pity coeds might have supplied. And *Inferno* gave us its magnificent mapping of the imaginary underworld's plan, with its circles or borgias, and its ordering of sin, which hasn't been attempted since, or at least until Michael Stone, M.D. produced a book and a Discovery Channel series, *The Anatomy of Evil* (2009), ranking criminal sociopathy to its hideous limits.

Rather than rely only upon my own judgment of what is funny about the *Commedia,* which is not about humor, I fortunately consulted David Dean Brockman, M.D., Past-President of the American College of Psychoanalysts, and a scholar both of psychoanalysis and religion (his son is a Monsignor). His psychoanalytic exploration of the *Commedia* (Brockman, 2017) could be deemed all you'll know about the *Commedia* on earth, and all you'll need to know. So I asked him, is *The Divine Comedy* funny? His reply follows:

"YES AND NO. The 'Yes' is that Dante was 'comedic' by stuffing Popes in maleboges (holes in the wall in Hell like burials of ancient Rome and of more recent time. And the only place!) The 'No' is that Comedy for Dante was derived from Comus and Oda (rustic village and ode song). He was writing this masterpiece to earn the honor wreath, but was never awarded it. Dante was less than a comedian with his clumsy and single effort to be humorous, and more out to get even for having been treated so badly by the corrupt religious leaders. He was a true intellectual and not so clever a politician when he went to see the Pope on an early mission. He got even with them by making them out to be fools in the poem, and stuffing them in the holes on top of one another. He wrote the first treatise on linguistics and etymology, so he was showing some of that in the poem. I see the poem as a monumental success. His only real effort at humor is when one of the many devils passes loud gas.

"The 'No' is: there is little else of equal humor. In the depths of Hell, Satan is frozen solid and his mouth is stuffed with various bad people including Brutus. You may know Dante was a famous diplomat who adjudicated a very serious dispute in Venice. He contracted malaria on the trip back to Ravenna and shortly after died there."

--David Dean Brockman, M.D.

For the purposes of this book, Brockman's reply to my query illustrates that, while classics are usually popularly entertaining and sometimes funny, their type of humor does not have to be at the top of our rankings--which focus on humor and not overall literary merit. The point of the *Commedia* is forgiveness and salvation, but the low humor of *Inferno* is unforgiving, sardonic, retributive, and cruel, ridiculing its targets (however much they deserved it) and wholly lacking in empathy. It can also be earthily gross. Brockman refers to the way in which Barbaricci ('Curly Beard'), a leader of military demons, signaled for them to charge: "...and he had made a trumpet of his ass" (*Inf* XXIv139,

trans. R Hollander). This contrasts, for readers of the poem with Biblical imagery, with heavenly trumpets. "*Inferno* is concrete and literal, *Purgatorio* moral, and *Paradiso* allegorical" (Brockman, p. 145). *Inferno's* humor receives highest remarks only in the universality of its address. For our judgmental selves that are fond of seeing failings punished, and large mischief punished severely, *Inferno*, like Kafka's stories about the system of his time, is irresistible because it is so exaggerated and over the top. The *Commedia* endures as the lambent canonical journey toward enlightenment that comes to mind with all other such difficult journeys, and is only placed down here because this is a ranking of humor.

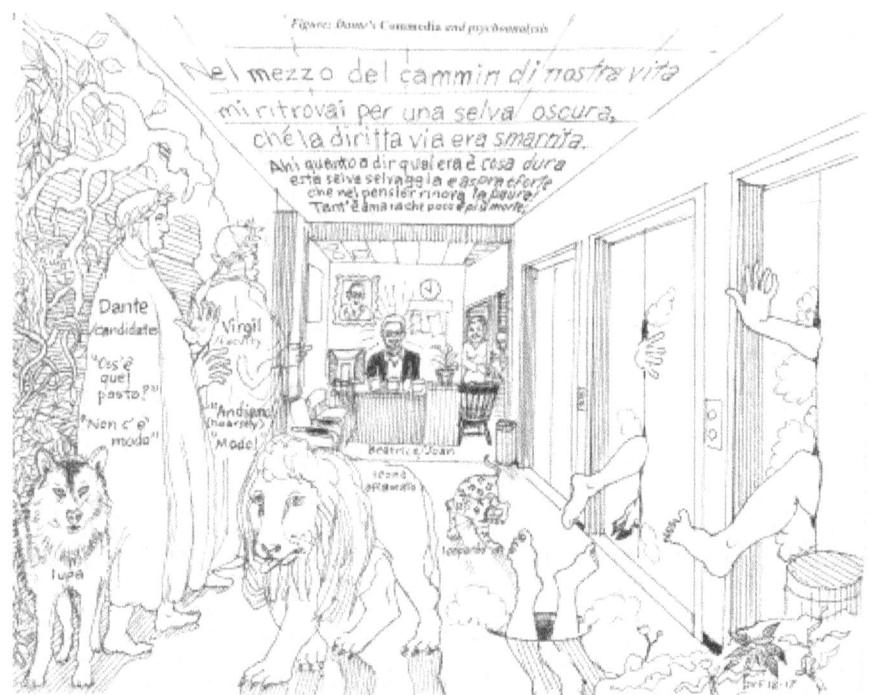

Figure: Dante's Commedia and psychoanalysis

A case in point about other difficult journeys being relatable to the Commedia is illustrated in the Figure, which I drew on the occasion of the retirement of Joan Jackson, our beloved administrator at the Columbia Psychoanalytic Center, whom I portray as Dante's guiding light, Beatrice. She is the welcoming figure seen at her desk. Also in the figure, Dante is guided by Virgil, who cannot lead him all the way to Paradiso because, as an ancient, he did not have the benefit of Christ, so Beatrice (also the Virgin Mary) must take over.

Portrayed as Dante, our psychoanalytic candidates' journey toward being able to think like psychoanalysts, and to apply psychoanalytic theory to therapy, the arts, literature, anthropology and many other fields, is an arduous inward one, both mental and emotional, fraught with soul-searching and many pitfalls, toward a profession Janet Malcolm called impossible (Malcolm, 1981).

We find it ever challenging and fascinating, but not impossible. Some have likened becoming a psychoanalyst and valorizing the tenets of psychoanalysis to religious conversion, but it is more like enlightenment, because it adds a capacity of thinking and feeling so useful that no one I have met regrets having acquired it. Practicing psychoanalysis demands extensive cognitive knowledge of mental development and defense mechanisms, and representation by analogy as in dreams; advanced pattern recognition and verbal ability; abstract and metaphorical reasoning, and imagining, especially of what is not being said. But the central element in the psychoanalyst's capacity is empathy, as was taught by Jacob Arlow, my own cherished psychoanalytic supervisor.

Mordant humor is biting, sarcastic, caustic, trenchant, and scathing. Edward Steed's *New Yorker* cartoons stand out in this regard, in the tradition of Virgil Partch (1916-1984). James Bond's murderous quips in the older films such as *Dr. No* qualify, as do George Bernard Shaw quotes such as, "Compassion is the fellow-feeling of the unsound" (*Revolutionist's Handbook*, 1903, p. 243.

Requires: a degree of liberty with, or controlled disinhibition of, aggressiveness, cruelty, or sadism.

Cynical/sardonic humor--Christopher Hitchens (2011) wrote about the "forced merriment" of Christmas as a time of "compulsory bad taste--entire families compose long letters of confessional drool." This is a type of humor favored by adolescents and the world-weary. (See quote from the theatre critic character described under **Burlesque**, played by George Sanders, who describes himself as "a killer").

S.J. Perelman, who published in *The New Yorker* in the 1930s and 1940s, wrote many sardonic and spoofing pieces about advertising (underwear), famous people (faux letters from Gauguin), fads (sleep masks, avocados), doctors ("osteosynchrondroiticians"), body functions (peristalsis) and best of all, himself, in his self-introduction by "Sidney Namlerep" ("in the verdict of history, the most picayune prose ever produced in America") (1947, ix-xiv).

Requires: An ear for sardonic tone, reversing meaning as in **Irony**. Some would say the acute perceiving of underlying truth.

Feuilleton (originally French, literally leaflet), began as non-political pages added to newspapers containing highly subjective cultural judgments written in a humorous, ironic style and employing devices such as parody, hyperbole and emotionally loaded wordplay. S.J Perelman had a feuilleton style, and more recently I would add Joe Queenan in the Weekend *Wall Street Journal* and Rhonda Lieberman (2018), who writes "Glamour Wounds" for *Artforum*. In addition to witty and often trenchant characterizations of contemporary artists (e.g.,"[Marina] Abramovic, where irony goes to die"), Lieberman delights with an un-self-conscious Jewish self-awareness, modeling a good-natured, interactive lack of sensitivity that the world now needs.

Commedia dell'arte was an important form of low comedy, court jester humor, and slapstick of 16th and 17th Century-Renaissance Italy, performed by a traveling troupe. Scenarios were improvised that employed stock characters with identifying masks, such as *zannis* (clowns), *Pulcinella, Scaramuccia, Capitano, Dottore, Pantalone, the Innamorati* (lovers) and *Arlecchino.* The story engine was the amorous intrigue of the *Innamorati* (lovers). Acrobats performed and made obscene gestures. Topical themes of satirical humor were woven in and adapted to the locale of the itinerant show. *Commedia* was the remote predecessor of low music hall burlesque, slapstick and vaudeville of the 1920s and later; and of the Marx Brothers and Charlie Chaplain. It was also the archetype for Shakespearean characters, classical ballet figures, and even sitcoms in which stock characters never learn, but love triumphs.

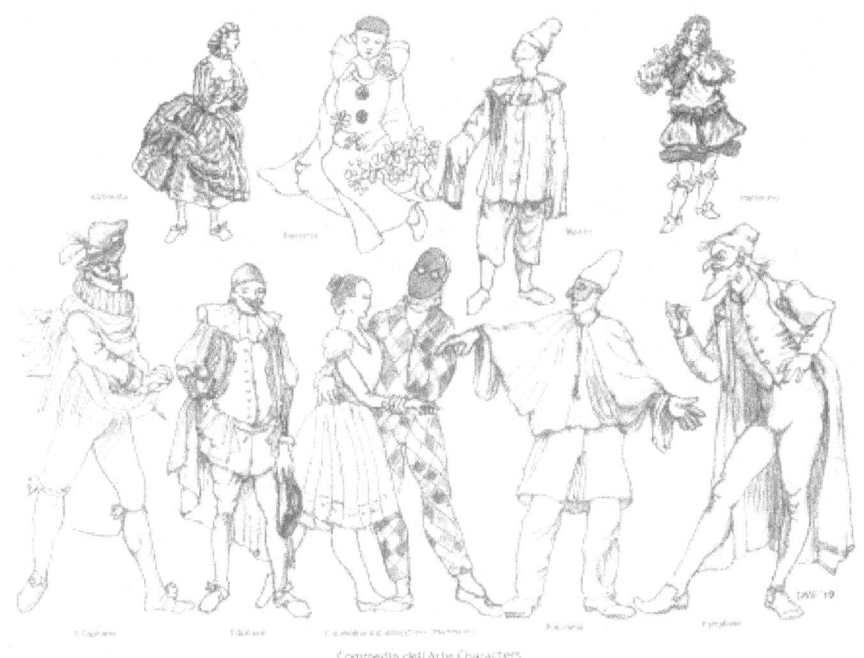

Figure: Stock characters of the Commedia dell'arte.

The Inamorato and Inamorata are the classy young lovers, costumed in the finest silks, who do not wear masks like the others, and lean forward as they move, as if literally falling in love, on tiptoe barely in contact with the ground. Their love is impeded by the vecchi, or old and parental characters, who are lampooned for the character flaws they embody. Il Capitano is a swaggering and bragging Spaniard, Il Dottore has studied all his life and learned nothing, Pulcinella (later Punch of Punch and Judy), is scoliotic and shaped like a chicken, and Pantalone is a greedy merchant of Venice. Other younger characters are the zanni, or clowns, who are servants of the vecchi. They include Pierrot and Pierrette, in sad whiteface instead of masks, and the gymnastic trickster Arlecchino (Harlequin), whose patchwork garb became stylized into diamonds, and whose stick begat slapstick. He loves Columbina, and they persist in Balanchine's ballet, Harlequinade.

Requires: Knowledge of the conventions of the stock characters and the topical issues and people lampooned.

Camp was on everybody's lips as the Metropolitan Museum of Art Gala on May 6, 2019 heralded their exhibition entitled "Camp: Notes on Fashion," echoing the "Notes on Camp" essay by Susan Sontag (1964, 2018) as "the love of the unnatural of artifice and exaggeration." Camp has had many definitions but exaggeration, usually outrageous, is common to them, and exaggeration is a basic comedic distortion discussed at the outset of these rankings. About camp at the Met show, Shaye Weaver (2019) wrote "it was first a French verb (to 'flaunt' or 'posture'), then an adjective with a gay connotation in the 18th Century, and most recently a noun to describe exaggerated gestures and actions. Notable practitioners of camp are the talented Lady Gaga, shedding layers at the Gala, Bjork, and the female-impersonating Les Ballets Trockadero de Monte Carlo. A follow-up article by Madison Mainwaring (2019) extended the umbrella of camp to all ballet, referencing Sontag, who included Aubrey Beardsley, Tiffany Lamps, Flash Gordon and *Swan Lake*, citing its codification in the court of the dancing king Louis XIV, its jeweled costumes, and fantastical characters, all of which can be campy.The argument to include ballet is weaker if one moves from staged royal extravagance to consider leotard-and-tights ballets, and the men's tights and tunics. The point of ballet as epitomized by George Balanchine is the incomparable beauty of body and movement, the strenuous athleticism and musicality required, and the devotion to expressing the score, none of which is funny nor played for laughs--unless it is intentionally camped up as by Jerome Robbins' in *The Concert* or by the Trocs (see **Physical comedy** below).

    Burlesque was lately epitomized by the 7th Annual *Menorah Horah* holiday burlesque show at Le Poisson Rouge, 158 Bleecker Street (the former Village Gate) New York City, December 5th, 2013. I was invited there by two of the fine arts models who participated in my previous book (Forrest, 2017), and found myself the eldest by about two generations in a packed house. Contemporary burlesque is having a renaissance and is more clever and winking than it once was, aimed at a younger, hip audience, and incorporating mime, music, puns and racy jokes around body references and disrobing (stripping). Stylistic references abound, such as the swank and slinky costumes of mid-20th Century performers, and there may be an element of épater la bourgeoisie, like presenting the Statue of Liberty disrobing. Other examples are *Les Ballets Trockadero de Monte Carlo*, "The World's Foremost All-Male Comic Ballet Company," Sid Caesar and Imogene Coca's ethnic characters, and John Belushi's "Samurai Delicatessen" (January 1, 1976) on *Saturday Night Live*. Burlesque is ranked lower in comedic acting, so that in the film *All About Eve* (1950) Birdie (Thelma Ritter), a former burlesque player, is the maid to star actress Margo Channing (Bette Davis). Miss Casswell (a relatively unknown Marilyn Monroe) is described in cynical dry wit by the theatre critic character Addison Will (George Sanders) as "a graduate of the Copacabana School of Dramatic Art" (i.e., a showgirl).

Hilarody is a form of Greek mime that burlesqued tragedy. It has nothing to do with Hillary Clinton.

Requires: appreciation of styles and conventions of the referents of takeoffs, and a sense of absurdity beyond literalness. Sufficient mental distance is needed to experience the eroticism in its intended context, and not just directly.

Lampoon is a harsh satire often directed at an individual (Shaw, Cuddon). Alexander Pope's *Epistle to Dr. Arbuthnot* (1735): "You think this cruel? take for a rule/ No creature smarts so little as a fool." Other examples could be drawn from *The Harvard Lampoon* (1876-), *National Lampoon* (1970-), *The Onion* (1988-), or *The Princeton Tiger* (1882-), which severely satirized Brooke Shields in 1983. Lampoons may be considered over-the-top personalized parody.

Another lampoon category is jokes that exaggerate and ridicule the characteristics of public figures. An example:

Donald Trump, Vladimir Putin, and Kim Jong Un walk into a bar [Some might say that's enough of a joke, and the listener could fill in the rest].

Trump orders a diet coke, Putin Russian vodka, and Kim also Russian vodka [yes, that's what he now drinks].

Putin starts the bragging: We Russki poot man in space in 1961, our Yuri Gagarin.

Trump: If you say so, Bro! But a lot of people have told me America put a man on the *moon* in 1969, our Neil Armstrong! How about you, Little Rocket Man?

Kim: Not to call me Little Rocket Man! Soon North Korea send *big* rocket, put army on *sun*!

Putin: Russki science, best in vorld, say sun *too hot* for cosmonauts.

Kim: Hokay! Then we do it at night!

Trump: Ooh! That's so fake! Believe me, everybody knows, and you can trust me on this, folks, there's no sun at night!

Requires: as in caricature, the ability to perceive unique and idiosyncratic quirks in the mannerisms of the people targeted. An ear for impressions of tone and accent helps, when the imitated group is not thought offensive to imitate (because historically less the target of prejudice). For example, in the above joke, reversing Rs and Ls in imitating an Asian would not have been acceptable, but imitating a Russian accent is probably less risky. Jokes in offensive accents are ranked lower in empathy, as put-downs. Examples are faux or obscene fortune cookie proverbs, for examples, "Man who sleep on back wake with jellyfish on stomach." The perennial "Help, I'm a prisoner in a fortune cookie factory" is sophomoric. Imitation is no longer always the sincerest form of flattery, as the saying went. See **Ethnic humor** below.

Travesty is an absurd, distorted or grotesque parodic imitation, as in Sasha Baron Cohen's *Borat,* a 2006 British-American mockumentary film portrayal of Kazakhstan; or the 2016 film, *Sense and Sensibility and Zombies.* Often it is of much lower quality than the original. *The Death of Stalin,* the brilliant 2018 film by Armando Ianucci (See **Farce**, above) was deemed a travesty by Putin's proudly sensitive Russia.

Requires: Blunt grasp of the characteristics of the chosen targets and the ability to relate the distortions to them.

Blunder is stumblebum physical humor, including pratfalls, e.g., Chevy Chase's elaborate falls, or Mary Katherine Gallagher's backward flops showing her underwear (Molly Shannon on *Saturday Night Live*), and Chris Farley as an overweight (but mostly surprisingly graceful) figure skater. It can be debased to a cruel ridicule of challenged persons; for example, tricks played on a blind man on stage. A more refined example is the Mistake Waltz in Jerome Robbins' ballet *The Concert,* in which one unfortunate ballet dancer of six keeps getting out of sync..

Requires: Comprehension of the deviance from the proper comportment, physical manners, or elements of the art humorously portrayed; crude ability to enjoy fails.

Dark /Gallows/Morbid humor /Black humor/Dark comedy. Examples are Charles Addams' cartoons, Virgil Parch, Dark Clowns (see Jason Zinoman, The tears and fears of a clown, *The New York Times, The Arts,* pp. C1, C2). Disrespectful graveyard and anatomy lab humor is frowned upon. George Romero's film *Night of the Living Dead* and other popular horror series employ humor, e.g. "They don't move fast. They're dead, you know." Often horror films feature a sequence of murders of victims who exhibit minor naive traits or behaviors the adolescent audiences find annoying. The victims are dispatched in a sardonic manner. **James Bond's Humor,** especially in the early films, involved insouciant killings accompanied by ironic statements or puns. Black Humor was earlier called **Gallows Humor.** John Donne, the Metaphysical 17th-Century poet, grotesquely wrote "Go and catch a fallen star/ Get with child a mandrake root." The mandrake was said to grow under gallows, and hanged men were said to ejaculate reflexively, so Donne is suggesting two impossible tasks, that is, catching a shooting star and impregnating the mandrake plant with the semen of the hanged man. The Metaphysical poets loved being jarring.

Requires: An ability to distance oneself intellectually from morbidity and death with bravado or insouciance.

Freud's jokes- are placed here after **Black humor** with ethnic humor. As a recipient of prejudicial treatment as a mem-

ber of the Jewish minority by his Viennese society and its medical community, Freud's examples of humor with which he populated his theories (Freud, 1905, 1928) were neither happy nor fun, aside perhaps for his description of freudian
slips. He postulated jokes about others as scapegoats that were not cruel ("innocuous," "non-tendentious") but had difficulty thinking of any. His "tendentious" jokes are those that have a victim. Freud thought jokes safely packaged hostility or cynicism or sexuality arising from the depths.

Word plays "condensed" conscious and unconscious elements. Jokes about oneself avoided horror in a "triumph of narcissism, the ego's victorious assertion of its own invulnerability" (Humor, p. 217). His example is "a criminal is being led to the gallows on a Monday and observes, 'Well, this is a good beginning to the week'" (p. 215). Such joking is common in countries whose citizens feel politically oppressed. Also akin are Franz Kafka's stories, which were deemed hilarious and satirical at the time, but belong higher in this hierarchy along with satire, because they required social and political consciousness of a "Kafkaesque" bureaucracy.

Jewish comedy and jokes--Although Jewish humor has its unique cachet, as a level it typically shares the rueful irony of oppressed underdogs discussed above regarding Freud. Jeremy Dauber (2017) in an authoritative scholarly treatment considers Jewish comedy under 7 headings: (1) responses to anti-Semitic persecution, (2) Jewish society satire, (3) wit, (4) crude humor, (5) metaphysical irony, (6) Jewish folk humor, and (7) attempts to define Jewishness. Cathleen Schine (2017), in her review of Dauber's book, chooses a joke from the pogrom era: "Two Jews before a Russian firing squad, both offered blindfolds. One accepts, the other scornfully refuses. His friend urges him: 'Shhh...don't make trouble.'" Schine writes that a black, Muslim, or gay comedian could tell the same sardonic joke. It embodies a social dynamic in a way more straightforward than nuanced, and at the same time lectures against submissiveness as an inwardly self-directed orientation.

Hoberman and Shandler (2003, pp. 278-9) describe how the sitcom *The Nanny* (CBS, 1993-99) with Fran Drescher moved on from sentimentality and self-mocking of Jewishness as inherently funny, to subverting the social order and celebrating the heroine's *chutzpah* in playful assertiveness. The nanny's upper-class employer is British, so to the audience, the Jewish Nanny has now at last fully become an American.

The much-lauded comedy-drama, *The Marvelous Mrs. Maisel*, produced by Amy Sherman-Palladino (which premiered March 17, 2017 on Amazon Prime), is about an Upper West Side New York Jewish housewife who discovers she has a talent for stand-up when husband leaves her, and is replete with humor about Jewish attitudes. Set in 1958, it is a master class on comedy that references such comics of that era as Mort Sahl, Red Foxx, Jack Paar, and Moms Mabley, and has a recurring Lenny Bruce character.

Jewish humor is a subset of **Ethnic Humor.** In his Foreword to Wilde's (1978) *Complete Book of Ethnic Humor,* now greatly dated in sensibilities, to put it mildly, comedian and toastmaster George Jessel characterized it as "laughing at the language mistakes and idiosyncrasies of grandparents and relatives from the old country" (pp. xi-xii). In a word, ethnic humor is based on stereotypes, and almost all the examples in Jessel's book for 21 ethnicities are unacceptable by today's standards of political correctness. When told by a member of the targeted ethnic group and loving or not self-deprecatory, ethnic humor can be subtle, hilarious and acceptable. From the lips of an outsider, it is usually a **Put-Down**.

Imitation of the accents of an ethnic group to which one does not belong is increasingly taboo, but it is interesting that some ethnic groups remain more acceptably imitated or caricatured than others who have historical claims to discrimination. Similar inconsistencies also exist in the newly invented offense of cultural appropriation, and are worthy of more extensive consideration than is possible here, but they involve perceived status, victimization and oppressor vs. oppressed.

Jesus's humor - Jesus brought joy to the world of Christians, but no humor? Terry Eagleton (2019), who has written a new book, *Humor* (Yale, New Haven, 2019), assesses humor in the New Testament:

"Many a commentator has observed that, though Jesus weeps, he does not laugh.... It is true that the Jesus portrayed by the New Testament is hardly remarkable for his side-splitting sense of fun, having as he did a fair amount to feel glum about."

There's certainly not any Jewish jokes from Jesus, but the epigrammatic beatitudes are so ironically paradoxical that they might have at least some communality with humor--for example, "Blessed are the poor in spirit, for they shall inherit the earth" --Matthew 5:3.

Culture-bound humor is a huge subject beyond the scope of the present examination of levels of humor. All the anthropologists and sociologists of every culture on earth present and past could not exhaust it, even if problems of translation were surmounted. It interests me, because for several decades I attended annual anthropology colloquia with leading anthropologists and psychoanalysts and have myself published anthropological studies, particularly of Vietnamese mythology and child rearing. The popular cabaret theatre of a particular culture hardly reflects its subtleties. For example, Japanese cabaret features physical comedy, slapstick and puns. These do not reflect the stately subtleties of the *Noh* plays, which themselves have relieving 30-minute *Kyogen* satires poking fun at human weaknesses and high-class samurai patrons. Frank vulgarity in the *Edo* period gave way to more gentle wordplay in modernity. *Manga* and *anime* cartoons range from pornographic sexual themes to narratives of great graphic beauty and philosophic meaning. And then there is *The Tale of Genji,* considered at the top of this ranking. Often one culture will have jokes at the expense of another. South Koreans have North Korea jokes, for example, to "nuke the Chinese" is to microwave the takeout.

Scottish humor -- Hilde Pedersen, M.D., a Columbia Presbyterian anesthesiologist who was born and educated in Scotland, supplied me with a video of two Scottish men in a voice-recognition elevator trying to get it to take them to the eleventh floor, and getting no response because of their Scottish accent. Growing humorously more discomfited, they lose control, lapsing into a burr incomprehensible to the rest of us. As one climbs atop the other to try to escape, the elevator door opens, revealing this to an audience of people waiting for the elevator. The humor seems to be the progressive undermining of the legendary Scottish reserve, as well as their dialect. Dr. Pedersen also cited the 18th Century poem "Tam O'Shanter" by Robert Burns, which is often read aloud at gatherings in Scotland to much merriment, but when rendered in standard English is considered no longer funny. Tam flees temptation in the form of the lustful witch Nannie, in a scanty cutty sark (short shift or underskirt), who pulls his horse's tail off as he escapes. The ship Cutty Sark (for which the Scotch whisky was named) has a figurehead of the witch in her chemise holding the tail of Tam's horse Meg. For fun Burns wrote eight lines within the poem in contrasting Standard English. Otherwise it reads like, "O Tam! had'st thou but been sae wise/ As taen thy ain wife Kate's advice!/ She tauld thee weel thou was a skellum,/ A bletherin, blusterin, drunken blellum," and it *needs* to sound like that.

Dr. Pedersen had some reservation (personal communication, May 7, 2019) about my take on Scottish humor:

"I agree with what you are saying, but see it as a risky business. Representations of accents or dialects can be described in terms of indirect non-referential indexicality (not much humor in that), and are often intended to imply inferiority (racial or otherwise), lack of education, or, at best, the hierarchy of languages. ("English da best!"). Examples would be Spanglish, Chinglish, or, in a different sense, Fake French, where there is an assumption of greater sophistication or *élan* in the French. I don't think these usages are common in the descendants of immigrants from those countries. More relevant, it seems to me, is that humor has an "in" quality within a group, which is not readily translated. While some Scots speak in a dry, taciturn way, anthropologists would probably shy away from assigning 'legendary reserve' on the basis of one or two samples."

When I asked what was meant by indexicality, Dr. Pedersen elaborated (also May 7, 2019):

"Indexicality is what 'a thing is,' or thingieness. It is subdivided into referential (e.g. I, you, she, this, etc.), that is, referring to itself; and non- referential, that is, bringing in further concepts, such as an accent does. Mara Green [a Columbia anthropologist] thought of non-referential as 'eating up the world'. A blue ball on the table, is referential; whereas, a red EXIT sign would not just be a red exit sign on the wall, but would indicate that there was a door or window there, or further, that it was a public space, or that it was a modern, well-run building, or that red is more easily seen in the dark, and on and on."

I surmise then that Scottish or any ethnic humor is freighted with non-referential attributes that lend it context. One would need to be familiar with these attributes to appreciate them, or to load them with attitudes toward the group, which could be admiring or critical. The same is so with the dialects. Thus to summarize from the above:

Dialect jokes--The humor of dialects and accents risks judgments of offensiveness or political incorrectness, risks being felt as a deprecation or even a cultural appropriation, but it can be funny when tolerable. It is sometimes lovingly delivered by those in a later generation mimicking their own immigrant parents or grandparents with that accent.

Pidgin also is real language in the interface between linguistic groups. It is not intrinsically funny, but may become so when outlandish, as in Chinglish (Radtke, 2007), or errors by sinophones attempting English signage. which may be poked fun at or described in a deprecatory way.

Requires: knowledge of the language attempted, and often the purported attributes of the ethnicity. Ranking the humor involved necessitates locating it on a gradient of admiration, mere characterization, or outright deprecation--the last lowering the ranking because of brutishness.

Borsht Belt and *Shtick* humor is an often stereotypical Jewish humor playing on supposed Jewish traits of (list from Wikipedia) "self-deprecation, insults, complaints, marital bickering, hypochondria, wordplay, and liberal use of Yiddish." A comic's *shtick* is repeated bits of business identified with him or her (e.g. Rodney Dangerfield squirming and hooking his finger in his collar, or saying "I don't get no respect!"). Asked what joke he would engrave on Voyager to represent us to aliens, Jerry Seinfeld (Amira 2018) said a Rodney Dangerfeld joke was "about perfect:" "I was making love to my wife and she had a faraway look in her eyes. I said, 'Darling, is there someone else?' and she said 'There must be.'" Anyone's too-often repeated refrain may be called their shtick. It may be sacrilege to suggest Coleridge's (1798) "The Rime of the Ancient Mariner" is a schtick, but Hunt Emerson made the guilty tale into a comic book (Knockabout Comics/Eclipse Books, 1989).

Adult animated series -- These strike me as sardonic, potty-mouthed social satire for the post-MAD Magazine generation. They employ exaggeration and reversal of expectation, and the interpersonal dynamic is pitiless if not brutal. Examples of this animated genre are Seth MacFarlane's (1999-) *Family Guy* and Trey Parker and Matt Stone's (1997-) *South Park*. The 1999 satiric film, *South Park: Bigger, Longer and Uncut*, contained 399 swear words and 128 offensive gestures in 81 minutes, and the song, "Blame Canada." My teacher son Daniel Forrest (personal communication, October 13, 2019) described *Rick and Morty*, an adult-oriented sci-fi sitcom produced by Justin Roland and Dan Harmon for The Cartoon Network's *Adult Swim*, as "surreal, observational humor, with satire, wit and character humor. You are on the money with exaggeration and reversal, but I don't focus on the 'potty mouth' aspect, as this is common to serious satire (Shakespeare, Rabelais). As for the pitiless interpersonal dynamic, Aristotle in his *Poetics* said both comedy and tragedy require suffering, but tragedy shows us as better than we are and comedy as worse."

Put-downs, as has been said, include ethnic jokes (like Rastus jokes or Polish jokes), blonde jokes, moron jokes and the like. Self-deprecating jokes would be rated higher. But not Winston Churchill's famous but possibly apocryphal put down: "Yes, madam, I'm drunk. But tomorrow when I wake up, I shall no longer be drunk, but you will still be ugly." The *Big Bang Theory* sitcom's ridicule of physics nerds who have autistic social difficulties is a put-down. Most find this funny but some math and science people find it anti-intellectual and insulting, or evidence that our culture prefers the mind of a pretty actress-waitress to minds in difficult STEM careers..

Put-down jokes can be insulting, as for example in the **light bulb joke**, that is, how many of a certain category of people does it take to change one. The answer is usually more than one, and the other person does something stupid or cumbersome, like revolving a table beneath the person unscrewing and screwing the bulb.

Usually the answer is specific about the category of person, e.g., it takes a number of Californians so they can share the experience. It only takes one therapist, but the light bulb has to want to change. Once my office mate asked me to change a ceiling light in our waiting room. While she was steadying a chair for me to stand on, a patient entered and could not resist asking that one! As I share my commute with many in finance, I once invented a light bulb joke for bond salesmen: only one is needed, but the threads and the bulb move in opposite directions (like a bond's price and yield).

We are going lower here, so perhaps inevitably there are off-color light bulb jokes. An old friend and colleague told me two:

How many mice does it take to screw in a light bulb? Two, but the problem is getting them into the light bulb.

How many Californians does it take to screw in a light bulb? That's silly, everyone knows Californians screw in a hot tub.

French military deprecatory jokes left over from old wars may still be heard, for examples, "Why do the French plant rows of trees by the sides of their roads? So invading armies can march in the shade"; and "Why do French tanks have rear-view mirrors? So they can watch the battle." (Such jokes forget Napoleon, the Resistance, and all that great French marching music).

Such put downs often involve offensive stereotypings. Blonds have been (possibly enviously) stereotyped as getting by with attractiveness (a look-ism) and not being bright. The so-called "ultimate **blond joke**" has both the driver and the police officer who pulls her over be blonds. The cop asks to see the driver's license. Digging through her purse, she asks, "What does it look like?" The cop replies, "It's square and has your face on it." The driver finds a square compact mirror, glances at it, and says "Finally! Here it is!" She hands it to the blond officer, who glances at it and gives it right back. "OK, you can go," she says, "I didn't realize you were a cop, too!"

President Trump engages in sardonic nicknaming of political rivals, for examples, "Little Marco Rubio," "Crooked Hillary," "Cryin' Chuck," "Jeff Bozo," "Sleepy Joe," and "Pocahontas" for Elizabeth Warren's Native American claims. He often uses physical characteristics: "Little Rocket Man," "Pencil-Neck Adam Schiff," "Alfred E. Newman" Buttigieg.

His sobriquets are so usual it is remarkable when he does not give one, as to Nancy Pelosi, whom he was said to respect. But responding to her remarking that as a self-appointed "extremely stable genius" he should act more presidential, Trump said (Schwab and Moore, 2019) "I don't want to say 'Crazy Nancy' because if I say that you're going to say it's a copy of 'Crazy Bernie' and that's no good. Because Bernie is definitely crazy." She remained "crazy" through the impeachment. He nicknamed Alexandra Ocasio-Cortez "Evita," admiring her media presence, while deprecating her present knowledge. "Mini-Mike" Blumberg again is looks. Trump does not seem to favor other types of humor than the put-down. But he did once manage a self-put down while commenting on addiction, saying "I'm not a drunk. I can honestly say I never had a beer in my life. It's one of my only good traits, for whatever reason. Can you imagine, if I had, what a mess I'd be? I'd be the world's worst!" (Associated Press, *The Boston Globe,* Monday, October 01, 2018).

Requires: conceptualization of social position, and the supposed (or insultingly and unfairly imputed) characteristics of the people who are the target or butt of the put-down. *The Big Bang Theory's* jokes and humorous situations putting down its nerdy scientists require recognition of the portrayal of their autistic spectrum behavior as deviant; and the ability to grasp others' emotional states (Theory of Mind) that some of the characters seem to lack. *Schadenfreude* is the taking of pleasure at the suffering of others, and it is taken virtually by seeing characters squirm in sitcom situations.

Low ethnic humor not just puts down, but debases and is increasingly forbidden. In contrast, **High ethnic humor** classified above, whether directed at the teller's own ethnicity or that of others, *appreciates* that culture. It can demand a nuanced knowledge of comparative culture--even an ethnographic savvy worthy of the anthropologists of old, with the self-knowledge of one's own culture-bound perspective. Humorists who practice it walk a line of near-offensiveness, and the jokes that work in one context, such as a Broadway stage, may fail disastrously in another, such as a political forum (as Jackie Mason discovered with his contrasts of Jews and Christians). Eddie Murphy's black humor on *Saturday Night Live* from decades ago is still winning ("Home for the Holidays" and "Mr. Robinson's Neighborhood," 12/21/19). Gervais (2020) recommends jokes be "bulletproof" for 10 years.

Rating of 2: Cheaper shots, Tasteless, Sick

Caricature and Impersonation--For example, *Saturday Night Live's* imitations of political characters. Kate McKinnon has played Kellyanne Conway, but has deemed Hillary Clinton her "most meaningful" impersonation (*OK!* August 13, 2018, p. 72). Clinton was also impersonated by Amy Poehler, but my favorite was Tina Fey's impersonation of Sarah Palin. Will Jordan was best known for his full-body impression of Ed Sullivan, and said it was "a partial invention. He never said 'really big,' he never said 'shoo,' he never cracked his knuckles..." (Sandomir, 2018).

Political caricature evolves through a President's tenure by the graphic exaggeration of characteristic features. George W. Bush was more realistically portrayed just after 9/11 but with the Iraq invasion, Hurricane Katrina, reports of torture and wiretapping, and an economic meltdown, he progressively shrank with growing ears until he looked like a fly with large wings. Barack Obama's narrow head was much narrowed and his protruding ears were disproportionately enlarged, as was his toothy smile. Trump has become orange. One recalls that a principle of humor we considered at the outset lies in the discrepancy of comparison, or the exaggeration of deviance..

But as the saying goes, imitation is the sincerest form of flattery and need not be negative nor mocking. Adherents to the Christian religion try to imitate Christ in actions but also appearance. Thus one may see a young man with golden brown hair grow a moustache and beard for an iconic Nordic Jesus look, even though Jesus would have had "a broad peasant's face, dark olive skin and a prominent nose. He would have stood 5-foot-1-inch tall and weighed 110 pounds," according to a cover illustration and article by Mike Fillon in *Popular Mechanics* January 22, 2015 (which had appeared previously in that magazine in 2002). The historical Jesus's
face was conjured up by anthropologists and forensic facial reconstruction artist, Richard Neave. Other Christian cultures have portrayed Jesus with a black skin like that of their own people.

The point is, physical imitation can be based on a culturally determined convention, a socially constructed image, rather than historical accuracy about appearance, and is no less worshipful. A Facebook advertisement said to have been paid for by Russians with the intent of influencing the 2016 Presidential election depicts Christ arm-wrestling with a reddish Satan who is saying, "If I win Clinton wins!" while Jesus replies, "Not if I can help it!" (Nagel, 2018). The Russian giveaway is Jesus's beetle-browed, black-bearded appearance with Georgian cheekbones. America's heartland is viewed as embracing the Manichaean heresy that the devil is real.

I confess about my own identifications that I once grew a beard on a long sea voyage so that I could be photographed in the ship's library imitating somewhat the Jewish founder of psycho-analysis in Freud's famous pose in black tie with cigar. To be sure, this was cultural appropriation from a Jewish Austrian by an American Episcopalian--but meant as homage.

Requires: intact fusiform gyrus (facial recognition) and the functional sub-networks active in emotional face processing (Cao, et al., 2016), voice and language characteristics. Reading and being able to reflect back facial emotions is often inaccurate and inappropriate in schizophrenia, slowed and muted in Parkinson's disease, and not very fluent in the rigid methodical personalities often possessed by physicians and other scientists as compared, say, with actors. For this reason we produced a teaching video employing an actor to teach the valuable skills involved in *Making Faces* to challenged patients but also to medical students, nurses and other personnel (Forrest, D.V., 2014).

Practical joke--said to have been developed in its most ingenious albeit geeky form at MIT, where they are called hacks. In 1968 the students convinced *The Boston Herald* they had invented a shower nozzle that made snow. During the 1982 Harvard-Yale football game they inflated a black weather balloon from beneath the field with MIT written on it in white lipstick. Many pranks involved scaling the Great Dome of MIT's Barker Engineering Library, but in 2017 a prankster fell to his death. Three Princeton sophomores got an imaginary applicant, Joseph D. Oznot (= does not exist) admitted to the Class of 1968 (Wolfe, 2018), a perhaps better-than-sophomoric gag. If one wonders whether this practical joke exercise is worthy of the brilliant minds of these Ivy Leaguers, one may recall that the frontal lobes are not finished developing until age 25, a fact with which I have regaled students.

Requires: ability to appreciate the devising of technical components, and what is necessary to entrap the victims in a funny and often distressing situation. "Smile, you're on *Candid Camera*!" or Sacha Baron Cohen's undercover interviews, "Who Is America?" (Showtime Original Series, 2018), are similar.

Low Burlesque was typified by the seedier, less clever and more literal, old-fashioned burlesque, as in the Trocadero in Philadelphia prior to the 1970s. Contemporary burlesque is performed for a hip young audience and may employ sexual innuendo and stripping with swank nostalgia and purposeful satire. *Double entendres* abound, with one meaning risqué. It is considered a theatre art and not part of the sex trade by its practitioners, some of whom were fine arts models in my interview study (Forrest, 2016). See **Burlesque** above.

Requires: comprehension of broad humor and tolerance of the erotic. Contemporary burlesque demands a knowledge of its current and historical costume, style, and other referents.

Sick humor--Revolting and disgusting, sick humor seeks to offend by transgressing the most basic feelings or decency of standards. A *Time* magazine article of July 13, 1959 entitled "The Sickniks," named Lenny Bruce, Mort Sahl, Shelley Berman, Jonathan Winters, Mike Nichols and Elaine May, and Tom Lehrer as "sick" humorists. An example would be **Dead baby jokes**, for example, "How do you get 100 dead babies into a box?" "With a blender." "How do you get them out again?" "With a bag of chips." This represents a grotesque, transgressive violation of the universal instinct to preserve infants, and was claimed by folklorist Alan Dundes (1987) to have arisen in the 1960s as a defensive dehumanization of babies with second wave feminism's rejection of the traditional motherly role and legalization of abortion. The Vietnam War protest, "Hey, hey, LBJ, How many kids did you kill today?" was contemporaneous and may have been in part a similarly motivated displacement.

A far more tame, related humor appeared in the subsequent **101 Uses of a Dead Cat** (Bond, 1988). A preservation of the knowledge of social standards is necessary for the sick humor to be presented and perceived as ironic. Regarding sick jokes, Weems (2018) argues that being told we can't laugh makes us want to laugh. He cites repulsive *Challenger* jokes from 1986, 9/11 jokes, and thalidomide phocomelia jokes from the 1950s, such as, "What do you call a kid with no arms and no legs floating in a pool? Bob." He argues the latency before jokes about a tragedy become funny is about 2 1/2 days of grieving per lost person, so that the death of Princess Diana had a shorter joke latency than the World Trade Center. Weems also cites British humor researcher Christie Davies, who argues that the sick joketeller's intention doesn't have to be vile, and may intend to deal with incongruous or otherwise inexpressible feelings. People with disabilities who were better adjusted to them, and widows and widowers who had better adapted to their losses, laughed most at jokes about their disability or loss (Weems, pp. 77-80). John Callahan, confined to a wheelchair after a car crash that paralyzed him, is a darkly humorous cartoonist who depicted a posse coming upon an empty wheelchair in the desert. The posse's leader reassures the others, "Don't worry, he won't get far on foot" (cited in Kaplan, 2018). Callahan is the subject of a 2018 biopic movie by Gus Van Sant with that cartoon line as its title. I saw the first joke about the coroavirus epidemic of March 2020 on April 1. It was a Van Gogh self portrait with a surgical mask dangling from his one ear, and the caption "F--K!"

Ruthless rhymes and Little Willie - An early largely anonymous vein of sadistic humor that was a precursor of purveyors of dark humor about children such as Edward Gorey (1961, 1963) was the Little Willie rhymes that flourished in the early 1900s. My wife, Lynne Stetson, recited several she heard from her father. I found a *Little Willie's Book* that was published without an author or editor in 1911 by The Carol Press. Some examples follow:

Willie in his bright blue sashes

Fell in the grate and was burned to ashes
Now although the room grows chilly
We haven't the heart to poke up Willie.

Little Willie on the tracks
Heard the engine squeal
Now the engine's coming back
They're scraping Willie off the wheel.

Willie saw some dynamite
Couldn't understand it quite
Curiosity never pays
It rained Willie seven days.

Little Willie hung his sister
She was dead before we missed her
Willie's always up to tricks
Ain't he cute, he's only six.

Little Willie took a drink
But Willie is no more,
For what he thought was $H2O$
Was $H2SO4$.

In these grisly rhymes, Willie can be either victim or perpetrator, but the outcome is spectacularly ghastly.

Edward Gorey, in his *Gashlycrumb Tinies* (1963), created an abecedarian book of cruel fates for the tiny children of his title:

A is for Amy, who fell down the stairs
B is for Basil assaulted by bears
C is for Clara who wasted away
D is for Desmond thrown out of a sleigh
E is for Ernest who choked on a peach

and so on....

Requires: Conscious or unaware emotional detachment and willingness to tread upon socially established sacred cows, standards of decency and morality. Although this may be considered to be evidence of a character flaw or even of the autistic spectrum, emotional isolation in a person of normal emotional and empathic capability is a conscious or unconscious defensive process, requiring ego strength and psychic energy to ward off the emotional impact. This requires intactness of the mental capacity for suppression or repression, which is often lost in a variety of psychiatric disorders, including schizophrenia. Another example is what Robert Jay Lifton called "psychic numbing" in combat soldiers (Lifton, 1982) or, in another view, battle hardening. Hardening of the hearts of medical house officers is a temporary defensive phase in training, apparently unavoidable, but still regrettable, warranting mitigation (Newton BW et al., 2008).

Phallic jokes and comedy deserve their own category, and have always been with us. Perhaps the funniest example is the 1974 film *Young Frankenstein,* which Mel Brooks considered his finest. Spoiler: the Dr. Frankenstein (Gene Wilder) figure willingly trades his brains and articulation to the monster (Peter Boyle) in exchange for the monster's enormous *"Schwanstücker."* Perhaps erection is intrinsically funny in contexts away from imminent intercourse, reminiscent as it is of the awkward protruberances of embarrassed pubescent boys called to the blackboard at moments inopportune for them in front of their smirking classmates. A critic's pick for the best sex joke of 2019 (Zinoman, 2019) was Jacqueline Novak's meditation on the vulnerable and sensitive *femininity* of the flaccid penis.

Dr. Strangelove Syndrome - Speaking of uncontrolled extremities, in Stanley Kubrick's 1964 film, *Dr. Strangelove, or: How I Learned to Stop Worrying and Love the Bomb,* the title character, an ex-Nazi scientist, has an errant right arm that intermittently gets out of control, resulting in a Heil Hitler salute or inability to let go of things. Although grossly funny, this mimics the *alien hand syndrome,* sometimes called the *Dr. Strangelove syndrome,* which occurs as a result of strokes affecting the parietal lobe or in a rare atrophic dementia called *corticobasal degeneration,* affecting the opposite (contralateral) side of the brain. Aside from misunderstandings, sense of humor may be affected when the atrophy involves the frontal lobes.

Rating of 1-2: Unconstrained melodies

Screwball comedy--Examples are Lucille Ball 's *I Love Lucy*, Jerry Lewis's *The Nutty Professor* and his other work with Dean Martin as deadpan straight man, and Cary Grant and Irene Dunn in *The Awful Truth* (1937). Howard Hawk's *Bringing Up Baby* (1938), with cast-against-types Katharine Hepburn, Cary Grant and a tame leopard, is considered one of the best, not the least because of its cleverly written double meanings. Zany, goofy, wacky doings sans depth are typical.

Requires: a simple sense of how the character is messing up according to social or interpersonal standards, often by scheming or overreaching. Usually suitable for children and rather lovable (e.g. Jerry Lewis, by the French, and Lucy in *I Love Lucy* by everybody). *Fawlty Towers* (1975-1979 on British TV) with John Cleese of the *Monty Python Flying Circus* series (1969-1974), was also based on situations going awry in screwball fashion. Clowns are screwball.

Freudian Slip, Spoonerism, Blooper. The humor inherent in a person unintentionally making a funny error while attempting an unfamiliar language is usually forgivable, although it may be socially outrageous. I have painfully learned that it is possible to order beef in the six-toned language of Vietnam and, by getting one of those six intonations wrong, to order instead the waitress's breast.

While I'm recounting my misadventures, once at a lovely dinner in St. Anton, the snow softly falling outside, armed with some college German but little colloquial knowledge, I pointed out the window and attempted to say, "look at the little birds." Through great laughter I was told I had said "look at them having sex" (*voegeln* rather than *voegelein*).

Speaking of German, where would *The Katzenjammer Kids* be--the longest running comic strip, from 1914 to 1949 and still in syndication, written by Rudolph Dirk and drawn by Harold H. Kneer--without the German accents of the mischievous twins Hans and Fritz, who rebel against the authority of Mama, der Captain, and der Inspector? All ethnicities are not equally sensitive or protected, especially German.

Spoonerisms are often funny transpositions of sounds, named for the many made by Reverend William Archibald Spooner (1844-1930), such as "the Lord is a shoving leopard" for "the Lord is a loving shepherd." Freudian slips of the tongue are more meaningful verbal missteps that unintentionally reveal conscious or unconscious thinking or intention. Condoleeza Rice said, "As I was telling my husb--as I was telling President Bush." William Archibald Spooner (1844-1930) said "the weight of rages will press hard upon the employer instead of "rate of wages") (Wikipedia). They are often a mispronunciation involving a reversal in sounds arising from anticipation and resulting in a blooper. Thus Harry von Zell in 1931 introduced Herbert Hoover as "our new President, Hoobert Heever."

CBS-TV anchor newsman Jeff Glor (see Top Ten Live TV Freudian Slips, August 30, 2008, uploaded by Sai Basabu), speaking of poor-fitting condoms in India, said "the number of HIV in-*fuc*tions is skyrocketing."

Disclosure: Glor once generously interviewed me on CBS.com about my then-new book about machine gambling, *SLOTS: Praying to the God of Chance* (Forrest, 2012), and internet interviews are forever. Barack Obama, at a DNC fundraiser in Hollywood, June 19, 2015, said, "We should be reforming our criminal justice system in such a way that we are not incarcerating nonviolent offenders in ways that render them incapable of getting a job after they leave *office* " [he meant prison].

Contending for the most freudian of all freudian slips was the error made many decades ago by a typist at the psychoanalytic clinic where I trained and am a faculty member. She was trying to announce a discussion of Freud's article, "Some Psychical Consequences of the Anatomical Distinction Between the Sexes" (*Standard Edition* 19:245-258, edited by Strachey, Hogarth Press, 1925, reprinted Vintage 1999), which described castration anxiety. Instead she typed "...Anatomical Destruction Between the Sexes."

Requires: ability to reconstruct what was intended, and how the slip reveals repressed unconscious wishes that are condensed in the slip. See **Punning.** The errors that may arise in posterior aphasias are usually benign errors.

Wisecracks, Yo Mama, The Dozens--trash-talking someone in a verbal duel, for example, "Hey, nice pants, does your Momma know they're missing?" (see Jolie A. Doggett, *Essence*, 2/26/15), or the classic, "Your Momma wears Army boots." It is African-American in origin., and comedic.

Requires: Appreciation of the sequence of compliment then switch, pulling the rug out. Frequently it's in the tone and the rapidity of delivery, which is aggressively challenging.

Shaggy Dog Stories are a purposely long and circumstantial telling of meaningless elements that eventually fizzles out and disappoints the listener's expectation by denying a unifying and funny punch line. Sometimes the ending is obvious, like "the dog's not that shaggy," after a repetitious buildup raising expectations of how shaggy the dog was, so to speak. Another famous example (according to Berman, 2014) is Arlo Guthrie's "Alice's Restaurant," an anti-Vietnam War song which has nothing to do with the restaurant except for the chorus, and relates amplified events on and on. Extraneous and irrelevant elements may accrete in a shaggy dog story. I think also of the Ella Fitzgerald and Louis Armstrong song "Frim Fram Sauce" in which the singer rejects all sort of usual food and ends by wanting "the ussinfay with the frim fram sauce and chifafa on the side." Flip Wilson did a long story about a man who returns home to find his house burned down. He is told it was from a candle, and when he asks what candle, is told it was at the funeral. And so on, each link getting worse.

Rating of 1: Lowest forms, Callow, Sophomoric, Puns

Gags/One liners/Pick up lines--"Take my wife--please!"--Henny Youngman. "Are you from Tennessee? Because you're the only ten I see" (rating women 1-10). "When God sneezed, I didn't know what to say."

Requires: Willingness to laugh at very little, brevity. Some young men believe pick up lines do the trick.

Low Comedy--Knock knock jokes, which could also belong under **Juvenile,** for examples, Knock knock/ Who's there?/Atch/Atch who?/ God bless you! Knock knock/Who's there?/Olive/Olive who?/Olive you [I love you]. Knock knock/ Who's there?/Broccoli/Broccoli who?/Broccoli doesn't have a last name, silly! Knock knock/Who's there?/Dwayne/Dwayne who?/Dwain the tub, Mom, we're dwowning). This last makes fun of a speech impediment immaturity or disability.

The low British comedy of Rowan Atkinson as Mr. Bean (in his 1997 movie, Bean), as in **Screwball** (above), turns the ordinary into moments of excruciating embarrassments, and is not for everyone. Some find it tiresome.

Requires: Recognition of homonymic substitutions, polysemy (multiple meanings of a word; approximately 40% of English words have more than one meaning.

Schizophrenic persons, because of inattention or lacking a good feel for contexts, sometimes take the wrong polysemic fork, so their intended meaning is derailed by language links or other loose associations (Forrest, 1976).

Juvenile/Sophomoric--The cognitive psychologist Jean Piaget (1962) described a *sensorimotor* stage of early childhood (0-2 years), when awareness of the permanence of objects (things, other people) is attained. Even at this time, infants recognize incongruity. In the *preoperational/egocentric* stage (2-4 years), incongruities can be verbalized and played with (for example, mislabeled). In the (still) *preoperational/intuitive* stage (4-7 years), which is semilogical, a child can create nonsense words, pictures and rhymes, and intentionally mispronounce a mispronunciation. They may regularize word forms based upon deep linguistic structure rules, for example, "Kansas City *Chieves*" instead of "Chiefs" (as with *thieves* as the plural of *thief*). By the stage of *concrete operations* (age 7-11), greater objectivity and logical reasoning permit abstract, implied and multiple meanings, so a child can explain why things are funny. Finally, with the stage of *formal operations* (11-15 years), abstract thinking and greater realism allow a child to appreciate the structure of humor and the motivations behind it. The psychoanalyst Charles Sarnoff (1976) assessed that fantasy interpenetrates with reality until about age 8 1/2.

Compassionate doctors, nurses and dentists equipped with a guide to these stages can use humor to break the ice with their small patients. Darling (2002) compares Piaget's (1962) cognitive stages of child development with the stages of humor development proposed by McGhee's (1978). Because incongruity can be perceived and seen as funny by even young children, a doctor can propose to listen to the child's heart, but place the stethoscope on their forehead; or discover imaginary animals in the child's ear (or a quarter secreted in one's hand's anatomical snuff box); or even propose a fantastical etiology, like "did you kiss a turtle?"

Memes for teens and the future of humor - One clue to the future of humor might be what young people, specifically teenagers, laugh at. So in August 2019 I asked an 18-year old British youth and his girlfriend about what they found funny. "Memes," he said, without deliberation. What? I was familiar with the term invented by Richard Dawkins in his 1976 book, *The Selfish Gene,* to note a cultural replicator analogous to the gene, the biological replicator. The term refers to a unit of cultural transmission, and derives from a Greek word (mimema) meaning something imitated or copied. Now this young man was no fool. He was bound for Cambridge to study math, already had his own math program on YouTube (HarryDoesMaths) and could rattle off a bestiary of quarks. He was what the British call clever. Why was he interested in memes, and what could memes have to do with humor? He gave an example of an ad for a child's game ironically relabeled "everybody wins with Communism."

Following up, I discovered that memes are now internet fodder. There are lists of the best memes of 2019, 2018, or 2017. They may be famous images, like Tom Cruise jumping on a couch (in 2005 on *The Oprah Winfrey Sho*w). But they can be almost anything. Two of the top ones are "the blinking white man" and "the distracted boyfriend," which is just a woman scowling as the man she is with looks at another woman in a red dress. "The honey badger" series of memes is also very popular. As the animal takes honey despite being covered by bees, the voice-over says "The honey badger doesn't give a s--t. It takes what it wants." We also see it

eat a biting snake to the same refrain. Pets and pratfalls ("fails") appear often as memes. What makes a meme desirable for the internet is universality (one of my criteria for top-ranking humor) and malleability (ease of altering for other uses). I might add utility and fungibility. As the social media platform Instagram has expanded, it has become commercialized so that behind-the-scenes meme factories now troll for cute posts to shape the content, because more sharing means more followers means more profit from advertising (Wells G and Horwitz J, 2019). The site TikTok has many clips of memes strung together by young contributors, with their choice of musical accompaniment. Frankly, to me they are often silly and trivial home movies, and not laugh-out-loud funny. Used similarly to emoji, they express emotions and attitudes when communicating. They are both more and less epistolary in an age that doesn't pen letters. But they are also a form of visual thinking, of imagery that the internet makes possible. I supposed this could be funny, if one yoked the right heterogeneous elements together. Feeling ever more like an out-of-it old wordy guy, I next asked my 10-year old grandson if he knew about memes. "Sure." He wasn't yet on the TikTok image format, like his 12-year old sister, but he used Gif. What? That's Graphics Interchange Format, pronounced jif, like the peanut butter, according to its founder in 1987, but often pronounced as in gift. Gif is a repository of short video clips that can be manipulated, as in replacing one head with another. A meme can be a gif, but gifs are usually animated. He grabbed his pad and showed me "The Adventures of Mr. Bird and Other Animals," a sequence of images he and two friends had compiled and pasted together that involved a hummingbird flying from left to right, then continuing as a butterfly and then Mr. Bee in a hive with lots of bees flapping wings and then continuing to disappear in a collision with a cartoon eagle flying from right to left with *Oof* (sic, a printed meme). A flock of birds follows the eagle from right to left. Brief appearances by human characters named PewDiePie, Dude Perfect and Laserbeam Ninja are interspersed, as are morphing portals from the video construction game *Minecraft* (today's no-hands-on Erector Set). The stretched comparisons resemble my own cartoon, "Who Can Fly," included as a static figure [above]. *The Greg Gutfield Show* on Fox TV frequently airs gifs to punctuate attitudes, but they are often not very related to the political satire. One result of such reapplying of images may be less precise humor (cf. near rhymes in rap).

A few months after I wrote this, by late 2019 the term *meme* became omnipresent in the media. TikTok, whch is a Chinese-backed social media network, had risen so much that there were national security worries (Li Yuan, 2019) and it had been banned in the entire U.S. military by January 2020.

Requires: facility with visual images, which can be selected or sought, or created. The breadth of reapplicability of a desirable meme plays with contextual utility, and is analogous to polysemy in language (an element having multiple meanings). Not very much abstract thinking is involved, because the process is so tethered to the visual images, and tends to be literal. It does not appear to require a mature mind, although mature minds may enjoy such picture play. Rearranging and altering memes resembles the processes of the dreaming mind, which thinks in images, as Freud extensively described, and can resort to rebus-like representations. The meme communicator may store a wealth of images, but the point of the meme factories is to make available a library of prefabricated images so memory is not required. Visual processing must be intact, and an ability to apply emotion and attitudes appropriately to contexts.

What future for humor? Maybe I am making too much of these visual memes as the communicative language and humor of the young and therefore the future. And perhaps I am underestimating their mental and neural demands, and therefore ranking them too low. What is transpiring on these platforms is new, involves its own skills and may evolve. But I do not believe that the imagistic language of dreams evolves, nor does it differ much among individuals of very different mental capacities. Visual thinking, topology perhaps excepted, is in ways tethered and constrained. Less verbal facility may come of cell phone and other screen use. Verbal language, like math, demands skills that are developed by verbal and symbolic education. A picture is both more and *less* than 1000 words. This is not to deny that film and TV have their own vocabularies.

Children's jokes, for examples (with a nod to my grandchildren) include simple riddles such as: Q: Why did the fish cross the road? A: To get to the other tide! Q: What's a pirate's favorite letter? A. He loves the C! or, R...ggh! Q: What goes up when rain comes down? A: An umbrella! Q: What do you call an alligator in a vest? A: An investigator! Q: What's brown and sticky? A: A stick! Q: What did Bacon say to Tomato? A: Lettuce get together! Q: What do you get if you combine an elephant and a rhinoceros? A: 'Ell if I know! How does a dinosaur pay bills? With Tyrannosaurus checks! See **Punning** below. Children also love jokes that catch up adults: Q: Will you always remember me? A: Yes. Q: For a year? A: Yes. Q: For 10 years? A: Yes. Q: For 100 years? A: Yes. Q: Knock knock. A: Who's there? Q: See, you forgot me!

Children's linguistic prehumor is meaningless talk that imitates the speech rhythms of jokes, much as infants' preverbal babbling charmingly at first includes phonemes of no known language, then reflects the speech rhythms of the ambient native language. Dr. Seuss (Theodor Seuss Geisel) dwells on the border of **Rhyme for rhyme's sake** discussed below and delivers deep lessons simply put for children.

Requires: Recognition of portmanteau (condensed)

words and sounds, homonymic substitutions.

Dad Jokes--These are tired, lame, stale, corny jokes, often involving puns, told by Dads to a younger generation. They elicit groans and poking fun at Dad for his old jokes. So why do Dads who are not demented tell them? They reinforce the separateness of the generations and reassure the children that Dad is boring and has no sexual or aggressive agendas on his mind (that psychoanalysts would consider an oedipal transgression). Mitchell (2019) elaborates and includes examples. I told my 10-year old grandson Mitchell's Dad (Grandpa) joke example: "Two guys walk into a bar. The other ducks." He said, "Yeah, Grandpa, it's a *bar*. I heard that one in the summer of 2016" (when he was 7).

Requires: The interpersonal social sensitivity to get that the intent is not to be humorous per se, but rather to reassure younger relatives that clueless Dad is harmlessly out of date.

Slapstick--(and other **Sadistic Humor**): The Three Stooges, Laurel and Hardy, professional wrestling, *Road Runner, Tom and Jerry* cartoons, Mark Sennett's Keystone Kops (1914-1920s), *Little Rascals,* and Chevy Chase's falls employ sadistic humor. *America's Funniest Home Videos* finds mirth in peoples' accidental pratfalls. Psychologist Steven Pinker (2011) has argued humans are becoming less brutal because of various civilizing, humanitarian and peaceful trends. I recall a sadistic joke in *Readers Digest* following World War II [date unknown] in which a group of British Cockney toughs were beating up their victim. After a series of damages described in the joke, one of them said to the lead bully, "Breave on 'im, 'erbie, and give 'im some of yer 'oopin' cough!" I cannot image that joke in the *Digest* nowadays. A 2019 Netflix documentary, *Larry Charles' Dangerous World Humor* explores the sense of humor of a Liberian warlord who eats charred children yet finds Bill Cosby's (1990s) *Kids Say the Darndest Things* fun; and of an alt-right white supremist who "gets" Charles' 2006 mockumentary, *Borat!,* about a clueless Kazakh journalist played by Sacha Baron Cohen. **Imitation of disability** can be scarily funny but potentially cruel.

Tim Conway (and indeed many actors depicting old age by Parkinsonian slowness and *petit pas*) or Jerry Lewis imitating spasticity, floppiness or facial grimacing are funny unless one is familiar with patients with those disabilities. I have even wondered if Lewis's outstanding fundraising for muscular dystrophy was reparation to some extent. I understand a stumbling, or even maliciously tripped up blind man was a staple of Latin American stage humor. On December 13, 2008, *Saturday Night Live's* Fred Armisen sank low to portray partly blind Governor David Paterson, one eye half closed, holding a graph upside down, staggering around the set and getting in the way. The Governor was not amused when he learned of it. Jordan Peele's creepily humorous (2019) horror film *Us* stars Lupita Nyong'o, who scarily makes her voice catch in her throat imitating spasmodic dysphonia, a neurological movement disorder whose sufferers objected to the film. Today's understandable sensitivities are evidence of a growing intolerance of cruelty, even if unanticipated.

Physical imbalance (postural instability or abasia) is immensely disruptive both to one's sense of security, especially in older people, and to one's feeling of solidarity in one's close relationships; and as such, is a ripe target for cruel mockery. It is evaluated by the Fahn Pull Test (see Appendix). Despite such cruelties, it is not always necessary to relegate **Physical comedy** to the basement of ranking. Some may require high levels of **Physical empathy**, demanding knowledge of a norm or ideal of excellence (as in the appreciation of ballet, that increases with one's exposure to it), or any athlete's connoisseurship of their own sport. One needs to have a sense of what ballet should look like to get a funny ballet spoof like Jerome Robbins' "Mistake Waltz" in his ballet *The Concert*, which also contains some low slapstick.

Buster Keaton (1895-1966) was the "stone faced" (deadpan) genius of classical physical comedy in the silent film era. He considered *The General* (1927) his masterpiece. His stunts in many films rival Jackie Chan's of recent years. In Alice Guy

Blaché's film, *A Sticky Woman* (1906), a maid gets stuck in a mustachioed kiss after being made to lick stamps.

Another example of physical comedy that might be elevated to the higher ranks of humor, because its execution was so poignant it bought a tear to the eye, was the film *All of Me* (1984), in which Lily Tomlin becomes the right half of Steve Martin's body, leading to virtuoso posturing and dance.

Requires: The neurological correlates may include capacities for implicit memory, and stored patterns in the basal motor ganglia and cerebellum. The function of the so-called *social brain*, a term coined by Leslie Brothers (Kandel, 2018, p. 38), is impaired in autism. It includes the superior temporal gyrus, which distinguishes biological motion from inanimate physical movement; the inferior temporal sulcus structures which read faces; the mirror neuron system needed for empathy; the amygdala, which contributes emotion such as fear; and areas along the temporal-parietal junction involved with *theory of mind* (sometimes termed mind-mindfulness). Again, this is the ability to realize that other minds are independent of one's own thoughts and knowledge. Presumably these memories and functions could also become impaired when a patient loses mobility, but I have had some clinical experience with Parkinson patients who have difficulty envisioning moving and outings, yet enjoy televised sports with family. Often Parkinson patients resist change, especially moving physically. The great physicist Stephen Hawking, immobilized by a slow form of amyotrophic lateral sclerosis, could visualize Einsteinian distortions around the boundaries of black holes; but could one with such a disorder still have enjoyed viewing with physical empathy the sports he played as a young man? I would predict he could have, as his *mirror neuron* function (see below in the discussion of empathy) and afferent motor system would remain intact even though his lateral efferent motor pathways, such as his corticospinal tracts and motor neurons, degenerated. Lending credence to this, in 2007, at age 65, Hawking took a zero-gravity flight in which he could free himself from his wheelchair and perform gymnastic flips. When ALS is also bulbar, social-emotional deficits in facial emotion recognition can be present. Hawking's theoretical excursions into cosmology remained spatial on the grandest scale, in contrast to those patients with Parkinson's Disease, who have difficulty with spatial relations and spatial visualization. Theirs is more than a purely motor disorder--as of the lower motor neurons in ALS--because their lack of dopaminergic innervation from the substantia nigra is more widely felt, and there are other neurotransmitter abnormalities too.

Cerebellar function is being recognized as surprisingly involved in higher non-motor functions too extensive to describe here, but even affecting the sense of humor. Nadia Amokrane, a clinical researcher at Columbia, observes (personal communication, February 26, 2020) what she calls SCA (Spinocerebellar Atrophy) humor, which can be crude and inappropriately sexual, occurring mostly in SCA2.

Nonsensism is primarily a British literary genre, and possibly a bit precious for some. Nonsense is best exemplified by Lewis Carroll's *Jabberwocky* (in *Through the Looking* Glass, 1871) with its many neologisms ("T'was brillig and the slithy toves....The frumious Bandersnatch") and Edward Lear's *Book of Nonsense* (1846) ("He weareth a runcible hat"). G.K. Chesterton considered nonsense and faith to have a kinship based upon their independence of intellect (*A Defense of Nonsense*, 1901). Children indulge themselves in it readily,
untutored. Nonsense preserves the syntactic and phonemic structure of its language.

Requires: preservation of syntactic language and the phonemic structure of the language that is the point of departure for nonsense words, and their pleasure to the ear.

The language disorder of **schizophrenia** may sound like nonsense at times because of the derailments of the train of thought by sound and the polysemic literal referents of metaphor, but it almost always makes sense to experienced therapists. This is a large topic others and I explored prior to pharmacologic reductionism, during the era of clinical phenomenological description of schizophrenia (Forrest, 1976). **Posterior aphasias** are marked by circumlocutions and in more extreme cases approach jargon aphasia, more like unruly gibberish. Pathological nonsense is less intentional, but still meaningful, despite losses in command of the language.

The lyrics to the previously mentioned song, "Frim Fram Sauce," written in 1945 by Redd Evans for Nat King Cole, are sung by a presumably ordering restaurant customer:

I don't want French-fried potatoes/Red-ripe tomatoes/I'm never satisfied/I want the frim fram sauce with the ussin-fay/And shafafa on the side.

While it is agreed ussin-fay is pig Latin for fussin', frim fram and shafafa have been more debated. One web contributor describes frim fram sauce as "the oleaginous goo of deceit poured over some unsuspecting dupe." But the nonsense allows the diner to refuse every possible serving until the last stanza, which ends with "If you don't have it, just bring me a check for the water," indicating having had no intention of paying in the first place.

Requires: Intact language function, appreciation of how the nonsense distorts, but echoes declarative language--much as doubletalk does. To appreciate the humor, it helps to have a keen ear for its cadence, tone, syntax and diction of the language being spoofed; less so the scholarly debates!

Technobabble--A special case of **Gobbledygook** (a word derived from a turkey's sounds) is nonsense in which known technical terms and elements are strung together, usually elaborately. Perhaps the best example is the enduring "Turboencapsulator," a technical description written by British engineering graduate student John Hellins Quick and published in 1944. A *Time* magazine article (Salwen, 1946) reproduced it:

"The original machine had a base-plate of prefabulated amulite, surmounted by a malleable logarithmic casing in such a way that the two spurving bearings were in a direct line with the pentameric fan. The main winding was of the normal lotus-o-delta type placed in panendermic semi-bolloid slots in the stator, every seventh conductor being connected by a nonreversible tremie pipe to the differential girglespring on the 'up' end of the grammeters." General Electric's Instrument Department even created a turboencapsulator data sheet and inserted it into the *G.E. Handbook.*

Requires: Intact language, but also sufficient scientific erudition to spot the ridiculous inventions, which may be realistic-sounding neologistic coinages. When delivered by a white-coated apparent expert in an authoritative tone and cadence, in video spoofs by Chrysler and Rockwell Automation (renamed the Retro-Encabulator), the mock earnestness is funnier. Other examples would be to cite a German medical article appearing in a mythical *Deutsche Gierschift und Krankschaft;* or the legendary Fortney Zorchtron gadget of *Mad Magazine.* While technical familiarity is required, the level of humor is low. Worth noting, jargon is a more general term for language with many specialized words that may be unintelligible to those outside a particular, usually occupational group. It does not have humorous intent per se. For example, "prison prep" for celebrities facing incarceration includes prison jargon for survival.

Ghostbusters, a 1984 film written by Dan Ackroyd, Harold Ramis and Rick Moranis, directed by Ivan Reitman and starring Bill Murray and classy Sigourney Weaver as a hellish vamp, mounts a preposterous premise and delivers pseudoscientific gobbledygook deadpan with unhesitating audacity. Not the least of its enduring ironic charm is that its villain is an Environmental Protection Agent.

Technical language with which one is not familiar can sound like jargon, or even absurd. Consider the following excerpt from the summary of a scientific article:

"Here, we report the experimental observation of the emergence of a Fano resonance in the prototype system of helium by interrupting the autoionization process of a correlated two-electron excited state with a strong laser field. The tunable temporal gate between excitation and termination of the resonance allows us to follow the formation of a Fano line shape in time" (Kaldun, et al., 2016).

Those of us not familiar with theoretical physics, more particularly quantum mechanics and the famous phenomenon named for Ugo Fano, might deem this gobbledygooky, and even funny. Or how about an article entitled "Wallpaper fermions and the nonsymmorphic Dirac insulator" (Wieder, et al., 2018)? One imagines a new kind of weatherproofing, even if one is among the regrettably too few people who know about Paul Dirac, the second most important physicist of the 20th Century, who named fermions, the small, light-building blocks of matter, which have only a half-integer spin, after Enrico Fermi, who described their behavior.

In a January 25, 2017 YouTube interview with Baltimore Ravens defensive lineman John C, Urshel, who is also a Ph.D. candidate in mathematics at MIT, Urshel told his favorite joke: "Why did the topologist's marriage fail? Because he thought arbitrary unions were open." While it's true in math that they are open (and not bounded), that's not the point; it's the play on the idea of an open marriage. This is **Word play** and it is a simple joke that requires a knowledge of higher math to appreciate fully. Most will get the joke without knowing what arbitrary unions in math are. The interview cites Urshel's math discoveries, and includes a funny interview in which Joe Flacco, his quarterback he was hired to protect, humorously says Urshel has trouble counting how many "huts" he says. Urshel also discusses his concussion, which for a time affected his ability to do higher math. He soon left football for the sake of his math.

The National Museum of Mathematics had an exhibition of math-related cartoons (March, 2019, reported in *The New York Times* of March 22, 2019), some of which were puns, such as Dan Reynolds', in which a lawyer-right triangle is telling a couple who are also right triangles, "Mr. Hypotenuse, I'll need you to *sine* this, and Mrs., I'll need you to *cosine*. I'll need to stop at the store on the way home for milk and bread, and, then..."

The wife-right triangle is thinking, "This guy always goes off on a *tangent*." This example contains two homophonic puns and a play on a word with a double meaning. The terms may be technical--at least at the high school level--but the level of humor is again rudimentary.

Psychobabble-My beloved profession, psychiatry. has been spoofed for proliferating meaningless terms and foisting them upon people as imaginary conditions. Our famous DSMs, or Diagnostic and Statistical Manuals, lauded for writing universal, atheoretical definitions to advance our science, are not really manuals, nor statistical, nor even diagnostic, according to researchers who say the categories do not yet 'carve at the joints' of real, terrible human suffering.

Doubletalk--related to nonsense, employs "sounds-like" substitutions and mumbling or swallowing syllables to thwart comprehension. Bogus words and phrases and nonsense syllables are inserted into otherwise sensible sentences in a rapid patter. In the 1930's, while performing on the Borscht Belt, Al Kelly, who became known as Mr. Doubletalk, bollixed up a joke and continued with nonsense syllables, which convulsed the audience. Other comedians known for doubletalk include Danny Kaye, Irwin Corey, Jackie Gleason and Durwood Fincher. Most accomplished, because he could also doubletalk in French, German, Italian and Japanese accents, was Sid Caesar. When done well, it keeps the listeners, even those who are familiar with the languages, straining to understand for a while before realizing they are being had. Fast-talking American auctioneers in cowboy hats chant barely comprehensible filler words such as "you are able to bid" to keep the hypnotic rhythm.

Requires: appreciation of the art of phonetic approximation of the sound and syntax of the particular language. In the case of Sid Caesar, it is not necessary to know the foreign languages, but it is even funnier when one does.

Gibberish--B.J. Novak has a delightful book of exuberant sounds for children to voice, *The Book With No Pictures* (Penguin Kids, 2014). A parallel is clang (Ger. *klang*) associations in schizophrenia. Babies' babble is gibberish, but it has a developing similarity to rhythms, tone and diction in the ambient tongue. Gibberish may be unintentionally funny, like older children's substitutions based on unfamiliarity with adult words, as in "Lead us not into Penn Station" for "temptation" or "I pledge allegiance to the United States of America and the Republic for Richard T. Stans."

Requires: Ability to distinguish semantic language from closely imitative phonemic sequences, to find funny.

Punning --referred to as the lowest form of humor, and one of the earliest forms of word play, the pun is based on homophonic "sounds-like" word linkages, or homonymic multiple meanings of the same word. It is a play on words, or *paranomasia.* An example of a homophonic pun is: "Time flies like an arrow; fruit flies like a banana." One of the most famous homonymic puns in literature is Mercutio's remark, after being accidently stabbed by Romeo (Act 3, Scene 1), "'tis not so deep as a well, nor so wide as a church-door [double meaning in Elizabethan times of a vagina], but 'tis enough, 'twill serve. Ask for me tomorrow and you shall find me a *grave* man." The pun expresses that he knows he is mortally wounded, soon to be a dead man. A recursive pun refers back to the start of the sentence, e.g., "A freudian slip is when you say one thing and think of *your mother*" [another]. Other examples of puns are many of Freud's jokes in *On Wit and the Unconscious*, and Benny Hill's word play. In Charlie Chaplin's film *Limelight* (1952), Calvero asks the question, "What can the stars do? Nothing. Just sit on their axes," a double reference to asses and the Axis (Germany, Italy, Japan and Bulgaria that opposed the Allies in World War II).

Sometimes extraordinarily smart people can delight in humor far down in the rankings, such as silly puns that lack any pretense of meaningfully clever word play (as in Shakespeare, above). The redoubtable American Association for the Advancement of Science (AAAS), which publishes the leading journal *Science*, decided in 2019 to reward its loyal members with a T shirt to cherish always. It is bright red and sports a spherical biological cell with a quarter cutaway to reveal cell contents, such as its nucleus and endoplasmic reticulum. But, oh no! The cell has a little face and stick-finger legs and hands, one of which is holding, yes, a *cell* phone; and beneath all this is the legend, "Cellfie." Got that? It's taking a *selfie* of itself. Let's hope this *sells* youths on STEM careers!

The Indian Hills Community Center in Colorado likes to post puns and double entendres on a sign by the road, for examples, "Irony is the opposite of wrinkly," "First restaurant review on the moon: Great Food. No atmosphere." "Tried calling the Tinnitus Helpline. No answer. Just kept ringing." The last one verges on cruelty, as tinnitus is no laughing matter, and causes much more suffering than people realize. But the favorite is: "When you're down/By the sea/And an eel/Bites your knee/ That's a moray! [Italian, *amore*].

Tim Federle (2013, 2015, 2018) has written a series of books about mixology in which the drink recipes have punning titles referring to literature. Examples are: Romeo and Julep, 100 Beers of Solitude, Vermouth the Bell Tolls, Fahrenheit 151, The Canterbury Ales, Lord Jim Beam, and Rabbit, Rum. Others of his drinks are Hollywood puns, such as: Ben-Hurricane, Titonic, Taxi Screw-driver, The Muppets Make Manhattans, and Indiana Jones and the Shirley Temple of Doom.

Recalling Ogden Nash's "Candy is dandy, but liquor is quicker," perhaps **alcoholism** is the commonest and fastest way to degrade the sense of humor.

Perhaps on the assumption that psychoanalysis, like one's umbilicus, has intrinsically funny aspects, cookbooks pop up from time to time with freudian puns. One of the best, by non-analysts (Hillman J and Boer C, 1985), included recipes for Charcot-broiled Lamb Chops, Erogenous Scones, Little Hansburger, Word Salad, Stekel Tartare, An Egg Is Being Beaten, Morning and Melons, Moses and Matzoballism, and of course, The Interpretation of Creams. Familiarity with the literature of psychoanalysis is needed for these puns. My security guard friend, Mark Gershon, asked me, "Did you hear about the psychiatrist who was arrested for Gestalt and battery?"

It's the lowest form unless you think of it first! But a pun's a pun, no matter how elegantly it is dressed up:

> A horse walks into a bar. The bartender asks the horse if he's an alcoholic, considering all the bars he frequents, to which the horse replies, "I don't think I am. " POOF! The horse disappears.

This is the point in time when any philosophy students in the audience begin to giggle, as they are familiar with the philosophical proposition of *cogito ergo sum,* or roughly, "I think, therefore I am."

But this would be to put Descartes before the horse.

The following is an extensive run of puns about the Pillsbury Doughboy advertising icon (adapted from various sources, including myself; original unknown, possibly Dave's Garden. 2007; see also funnybizblog.com):

> The Pillsbury Doughboy died yesterday of a yeast infection and repeated pokes in the belly. He was buried in a lightly greased coffin. Dozens of celebrities paid their respects, including Mrs. Butterworth, Betty Crocker, The Hostess Twinkies, and Captain Crunch. His gravesite was piled high with flours. Do-re-mi from *The Sound of Music* was sung by Josephine Baker. Aunt Jemima delivered the eulogy and lovingly described Doughboy as too modest to know how much he was kneaded. He had risen rapidly in show business, but his life had many turnovers. Not too smart a cookie, he wasted much of his dough on half-baked schemes. A little flaky at times, in old age he was nevertheless considered a roll model for millions. Doughboy is survived by his wife, Play Dough, his two children, John and Jane Dough, plus one in the oven. He is also survived by his elderly father, Pop Tart. The funeral was held at 350 for about 20 minutes.

Dickson (1984) compiled "a collection of groanmaker puns...from classic to contemporary" (a cover blurb), some of which resemble shaggy dog stories that end with a pun. A brief example (p. 15):

A professor of Greek takes his torn suit to a Greek tailor. The tailor looks at the pants and says, "Euripides?"

"Yes," replies the professor, "Eumenides?"

Another rich source of puns is any cover of *The New York Post*. For low-lying, gross indelicacy, it is hard to beat Thursday, May 31, 2018, with its cover heralding:

"The Other Big Ass Summit/Kim Thong Un pitches prez on prison reform/TRUMP MEETS RUMP/Reality star meets reality president in the Oval Office yesterday when Kim Kardashian lobbied President Trump to pardon a 63-year-old first-time drug offender. Pages 4-5"

And then there's the riddle, "Q: What is 2019 impeachment Congressman Adam Schiff's favorite seafood? A: Squid pro quo."

Even the formidable British *Economist* allows itself puns in its headings. In an article, "Funerals of the Future" (April 14, 2018, pp. 51-53) the headings "Stiff competition" and "The Green Reaper" appear.

James Geary (2018), in his book on wit, notes that Shakespeare put an average of 78 puns in each play, and considers them not so much glib derailments as the essence of wit, because they involve holding two simultaneous ideas about something. But as we have seen, all humor does that by exaggerations, comparisons, metaphors or contrasts with social norms, and with more subtlety possible with length. And Shakespeare's great puns, as in *Hamlet*'s graveyard scene, rely for their poignancy on the context in which they are imbedded, and amplify rather than derail the emotion for cheap laughs.

Macaronic puns (from the Italian *maccarone* for dumpling, referring to coarse peasant fare) mix languages, or mean different things in two languages. Getting them requires knowledge of the languages. As with technical puns in specialized language, the content is independent of the level of humor involved, and may be derogatory or even obscene. A famous unintentional Greek to French example from Xenophon, about having no hope of taking a city, when read as French sounds like it ends in "Elle pisse et fait caca." [from the Wikipedia article on macaronic language]. James Joyce was found of macaronic puns, and used this one in *Finnegan's Wake;* as he also did "And Trieste ah Trieste ate I my liver," which sounds like "Triste, triste était mon livre," meaning, "Sad, sad, was my book."

Requires: knowledge of the languages involved, metaphoric capacity, realization of the polysemy of words. As Freud described it, condensation of multiple elements is intrinsic to brain function, so the condensation of elements in punning taps into this. In anticipatory spoonerisms and Freudian slips there is an implicit acknowledgment of dynamic unconscious activity revealing itself. In the sensational media, such as the headlines of *The New York Post,* a knowledge of slang is required.

Slang and problems of translation - Emotions, especially strong emotions, sexual themes, and humor tend to be expressed in slang. For this reason, when we at The New York State Psychiatric Institute were charged with training State mental hospital staff who were almost all international medical graduates from an assortment of countries, we created a dictionary of emotional and street slang for them (see Forrest DV, 1974) to aid interviewing and therapy with familiar language beyond the formal King's or Queen's English they were taught in their countries of origin.

Turning this around, as discussed above, caution is advised in evaluating a non-native person's sense of humor with Americanisms. Our foreign-born doctors struggled with humor in our TV commercials when it undermined authority.

Slang is intrinsically witty because of its eloquence. The brevity of slang when it hits the spot and cuts through formal verbiage surprises and delights. Yiddish is especially known for this, because it has terms for concepts and types that are otherwise inexpressible in a single word, or even several, if at all. Try to find a better single word for *schlemiel* or *schlimazel, schmooze* or *tchotchke,* or even *nu.* Yiddish theatre has favored tragicomedy, "laugh as you cry," and productions of *King Lear* and *The Merchant of Venice* have brought together the love of puns and word play of both the Bard and Yiddish speakers, half of whom live in New York. But Yiddish is a historical language, developed by the Ashkenazi Jews in the 9th Century, that can express as comprehensively as any tongue.

Figure: *Quibbles of an English Major*

In a spirit of disclosure, were there not evidence enough by this point in the rankings that I was an English major as a premed, I add 2 drawings illustrating an English major's incurable and persnickety fondness of correcting language. The first depicts one of my pet peeves, the rampant failure to distinguish suspect *and* suspicious, *the latter originally deemed to require consciousness and sentience to feel it. I regret that on this point the train, or perhaps I should say the subway, has left the station, no thanks to the usage felons of law enforcement, including the New York City Metropolitan Transportation Authority, who warn of "suspicious packages" and adjure us, "If you see something, say something."*

The second quibble was a reaction to the pressure to rename the Princeton Alumni Weekly *even more gender-neutrally by substituting* Alum *for* Alumni *(October 14, 2016 issue). Laudably intended, this infelicitous solution struck me as bathos, and I drew my mental association to the mouth-puckering chemical salt, alum.* PAW *gratefully published it (October 26, 2016 issue).*

Insufferable snobbery though these cartoons may reveal, they fall low in our ranking of humor. They are based on fine points of language, and do not require the higher cognitive and empathetic operations at the top. Word power, that is, vocabulary, declines later in dementia, and may even increase in general aging, while episodic memory for (newly learned) facts, fluid (logical) reasoning, and processing speed may gradually decline (as described by Georgette Argiris, Ph.D. of the Yaakob Stern Lab. Neurological Institute of New York Grand Rounds, January 10, 2020). There are reasons why older folks love Jeopardy *(facts) and* Wheel of Fortune *(phrases).*

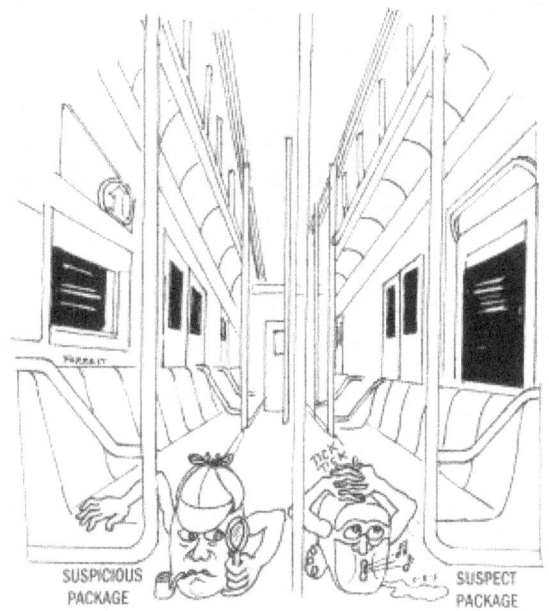

Figure: Quibbles of an English Major

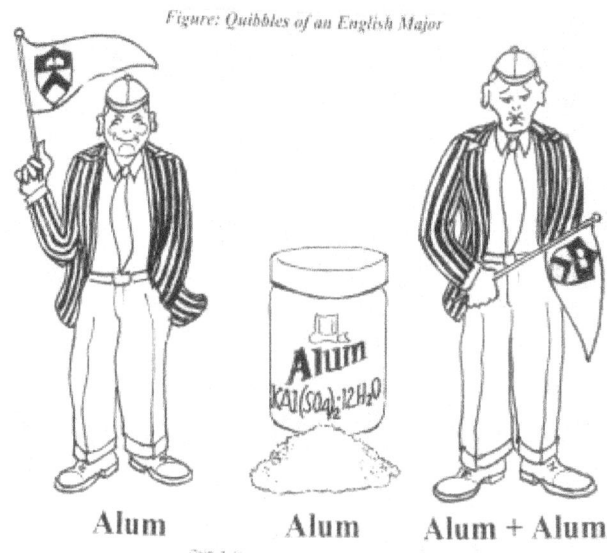

Alum   Alum   Alum + Alum

Rhyming for the Sake of Rhyming: Amusement from simple rhyming may occur in the *klang* **associations** by patients with severe schizophrenia; or in severe mania, along with overinclusive, kitchen-sink listing and punning.

Rating of 0: Meaningless Hilarity

Laughing at nothing: From here on, the focus is on the person who laughs, not the stimulus, which may be absent in:

Inappropriate affect of schizophrenia or psychogenic states, i.e., emotion incongruent with the idea being expressed;

Mania and delusional mania of severe bipolar states; the excessive activation and animation may make the humor seem pointless, not contagious, or too forced;

Gelastic epilepsy (with seizure-induced unprovoked laughter or crying);

Pseudobulbar affect lability (shifting expression like laughing, crying, cursing, et cetera) can result from some neurological disorders (such as multiple systems atrophy); the underlying sense of humor may be cognitively preserved;

Cataplectic laughter with muscle relaxation and even collapse to the floor, which may result from an emotional stimulus. The mirth is beyond what would be commensurate;

Silly laughter from cannabis or nitrous oxide toxicity.

Newborns are equipped with a reflex smile and at times it may just be gas, but as Jeffrey Pines, M.D. wondered to me, we don't always know at what babies are smiling. The stimulus need not be funny in any sense, and can just be a delightfully familiar toy or parent. The reflex smile gives way to the real social smile beginning anywhere from 6-8 weeks to 3 months, and laughing out loud at 3-4 months of age.

Witzelsucht [German for joke or wisecrack + addiction/seeking]: People with frontal lobe deficits may make jokes or comments inappropriate for the situation, pointless stories, sometimes without affect, and with inappropriate touching. Another term for it is Joker Syndrome (named for Batman's arch rival). Oppenheim coined the term *Witzelsucht* in 1889, based on Jastrowitz's 1888 *Moria* (stupidity) from right frontal lobe damage. Arthur Koestler named Foerster's Syndrome, for the compulsive punning that occurred in 1929 when the German neurosurgeon Otfrid Foerster manipulated a 3rd ventricle tumor (near emotional brain structures) and the patient burst into a manic stream of puns while on the table with his skull open. See Verplaste (2009) on localizing moral sense; and Kipps, et al. (2009) on understanding sarcasm, of which those with frontotemporal dementia may be less capable than those with Alzheimer's.

Similarly, the jejune cartoon characters *Beavis and Butt-head* disregard context and seek callow, raunchy, double entendres for their shallow, mutual mirth..

Rating of -0.5 to -4: Nothing funny for some folks:

Lack of a sense of humor--Donald Trump and his administration at times vie for this designation. Bill Maher, who granted is sometimes a bit hard to take, said he would pay Trump $1 million if he could prove he was not the product of an orangutan and a human mating. Trump and his lawyers produced his birth certificate and demanded the reward (which has not been paid). Maher's gag echoed Trump's having been a "birther" who denied Obama's having been born in the USA.

When accused of sexual activity with Russian prostitutes on a visit there prior to his Presidency, Trump failed to address the moral dimension of the accusation. Also abandoning any recognition of irony (which see, above) he first pointed out he was a notorious germaphobe, and then consulted Vladimir Putin as a character reference, who was also short on the moral dimension, attesting that Trump didn't need to solicit the services of prostitutes because he ran beauty pageants with some of the most beautiful women on earth. Further digging himself into a moral hole, and unable to resist living up to a Russian stereotype of boasting, Putin then bragged that when it comes to prostitutes, Russia has the best..

Lacking a sense of humor does not necessarily indicate a psychiatric disorder (which in our diagnostic manuals requires distress and unusual degree), or a neurological disorder (in the absence of other cognitive problems). It might be classified as a character trait, in which case it is likely to be permanent, or a temporary situational state. Last, it could be a posture assumed in response to shorter- or longer-lasting situations. If one is a frequent target of jokes (see **Freud's humor** above), one is not likely to laugh along. One needs to be free to laugh and not to be the butt of the joke.

Just kidding: This construction allows one to float a seemingly serious statement and then retract it. Hillary Clinton, speaking on October 8, 2019 to Judy Woodruff of *PBS News Hour*, said "There does need to be a rematch. Obviously I can beat him [Trump] again," and later said, "Just kidding."

Character types associated with a lack of humor: Rigid, controlled, *obsessive* personalities don't like jokes, partly because they don't like surprises or rapid shifts, which is what the punch in a punch line is all about. Their frequent smiles are without pleasure, and may be aggressive grimaces with an atavistic showing of teeth; or in defeat, a sardonic rictus of rue. *Paranoid* personality types also hate surprises, view them as sneak attacks, and are suspicious and fearful about vulnerability, so that nothing seems to be a laughing matter. They seldom laugh, and seem to cast a gloomy spell of ominous vigilance. Although not much fun, neither of these types are pathological per se, and each is good at certain things--obsessives, at exacting professions and paranoids, at watchful or judgmental ones.

Dramatic, *histrionic* personalities smile generously and charmingly, but may be given to laughing insincerely by way of flattery to give or win love or admiration.

Fortunately most people have mixtures of character traits, and most possess some sense of humor. But it can vary from a love of the absurd to pleasure in observing minor divergences from social rules; from the rueful and self-deprecatory to the cruel and pejorative; from subtle irony and trenchant cultural commentary to bringing up appearances or bodily functions; or from extreme wit to low puns and bathos.

Rating of -0 to -1: Targets of Humor and Butts of Jokes:

Once upon a time, it was commonly thought (by men) that women lacked a sense of humor. But the jokes women didn't find funny often targeted them. **Women** comediennes like Gracie Allen and Imogene Coca often set up male comedians, or were the butts of put-downs by the men, so they got second billing, like Ginger Rogers, who it's said did everything Fred Astaire did, only backward and in heels. Lucille Ball and Audrey Meadows held their own against Desi Arnaz and Jackie Gleason, but Carol Burnett got sole billing, and paved the way for such contemporary stand-alone, stand up comediennes as Sarah Silverman and Amy Schumer. These performers also have no trouble closing on punch lines, a hesitancy over-generalized to their sex. Although there are still many jokes *laughing at* women on the internet, I have compiled a list of women comedians to remind everyone how funny women can be to *laugh with* (see **Women comedians,** Appendix).

Rating of -1: Mourners and Depressed people, during the mourning process or depressive episode may understandably be unable to laugh at anything.

Rating of -2: Posturers adopt a humorless stance for the moment or for effect, or to impress others, and refuse to yield up a smile or be dissuaded from their righteous posture or claims of mandate. I would emphasize here that our rankings take no sides nor assign legitimacy or illegitimacy to any assertions.

Genealogy has another meaning than the study of family ancestry. In politics Devetak (1995, p. 184) defines genealogy as the historical study of the relationship of knowledge to power, "best known through Nietzsche's radical assault on the concept of truth and moral values in *Beyond Good and Evil* and *On the Genealogy of Morals.*" As such, the term genealogy applies to all changes in expression dictated by political power. As with the erotic, much humor derives from disparities of power; but power relationships can also quench humor (not to mention sex and love).

Some of the roles of humorlessness people assume, often

ad hoc, and *pro tempore* rather than permanently, include:

Police officer, judge, military personnel;

Political activist across the political spectrum;

Sanctimonious scold/bluenose/prude;

Censor, critic, cleric, referee or grade-giver;

Political corrector/language policer. The new so-called *cancel culture* of "throwing stones" and claiming to be "woke" by "calling out" people for language missteps has been criticized by President Barack Obama (29 Jan 19) in a widely-praised interview as "not activism" that produces change. Some of the woke have dismissed him as just another old millennial.

Psychiatrist or other therapist (who may laugh with, but not at, a patient's statement, even though it may be, by conventional standards, funny or absurd). A schizophrenic patient once proposed a bizarre invention for shaving: a concave device with whirling blades, into which one would insert one's face. This grotesque idea also concretely conveyed his problem with a flat affect, which was a symptom of his schizophrenia. I had to suppress nervous laughter at his deadpan.

Rating of -3: Zealots--and other true believers who may resist humor globally or specifically. May be political or religious zealots, given to extreme devotion or menacing.

Rating of -4: Victims and Lost Ones, Trauma and Brain Disease: Destroyed by traumatic neuroses of war or other events, their "ego turns to sand" (Abram Kardiner); or they may be burned-out drug abusers; deteriorated psychotic persons; persons traumatized beyond recovery, or those having had early profound deprivation affecting brain and behavioral development (described by Nathan A. Fox, Ph.D., regarding the Bucharest Early Intervention Program; Grand Rounds, New York State Psychiatric Institute, February 28, 2018).

Profound **dementia**, particularly affecting the frontal lobes, may affect the sense of humor. The apparent solemnity in **Parkinson's Disease** is a product of muted motor expression, and the sense of humor may be lively within. Persons on the **autistic spectrum** may force a laugh without contagious emotion, and at eccentric stimuli others do not comprehend or find funny. Persons with **frontal lobe disease** may laugh a great deal but fail to get humor because of deficits in empathy, working memory, and abstracting ability.

How to use these rankings to evaluate sense of humor

If asked, persons being evaluated or their families may themselves offer examples, which can be placed in the ranking as belonging to a level or analogously representing one. Prompting questions may be asked, such as "Can you think of a joke to tell me?" or "Do you watch any funny TV shows?" or "What made him laugh recently?" or "Does she laugh at funny things that happen in the family?" "Does she laugh at her own or others' failings or accidents?" "Does she get the joke when someone is just kidding/speaking ironically/being sarcastic?" When a person is laughing along with others, comprehension needs to be assessed, as opposed to just joining in mimetically.

To determine the highest level of comprehension of humor, it is well to begun at a lower level, or at least to adjust the early questions to the individual's probable level.

If a minus ranking for a lack of a sense of humor applies, one needs to assess further whether it reflects a
temporary attitudinal stance that might be mistaken for a permanent lack in the sense of humor, like a trait, or a brain impairment interfering with grasp of the humor.

The lowest positive rankings, given a rating of 1, may be tested by a pun, such as those about the Pillsbury Doughboy, for example, "He rose quickly in show business, but he was not a very smart cookie, and his life was filled with turnovers," or a child's riddle, for example, "What do you call an alligator in a vest? An investigator!" Dad jokes, slips of the tongue, or spoonerism like "the Lord is a shoving Leopard" can be used, but one must take care with any mention of religion or politics.

The crueler level of 2 might be exemplified with Little Willie rhymes or uses for a dead cat. Practical jokes can be asked about. One of the best was told by Alice Whitmore about underlings at her ad agency who daily substituted the boss's hat with one a size smaller and then one a size larger,

Level 2-3 may be evaluated with a visual caricature (realizing this requires intactness of facial recognition), or one of Freud's gallows humor jokes about a man in front of a firing squad telling another man not to make waves. One may ask about put-downs the person has heard, or obtain a reaction to well-known ones. Light bulb jokes usually have a targets and are put-downs. Ethnic jokes may be asked about, not quoted.

For each of these levels, some examiners may choose to make up a cards or a booklet of copied or clipped specimens of favorite humor to use in evaluation. But instruments of universal applicability elude compiling, because of the variety and limits of people's experiencing of stimuli. My many illustrative examples above at each level were given not to determine choices, but to convey the ideas of the levels for personalizing with one's own examples.

In all evaluations of humor, one would add whether it was a stable and usual fondness for a particular level, or if there has been a change over a specified time period.

The off-color level of 3 is best approached with care, or avoided unless brought up by the person being evaluated. The dignity of the examiner and the comfort of the person examined remain paramount. One might approach indirectly, not citing a specific specimen of humor, but asking about the person's interest in any off-color material, and whether there has been a change in interest. Certain dementias, mood swings, and dopamine-increasing medications can increase salacious interest generally, and this can be embarrassing for patients and their families. Dementia, apraxia or confusion can lead to false impressions of sexual intent, for examples, incompletely dressing or disrobing or urinating in the wrong place. The examiner can inquire about milder off-color examples such as limericks. If the sense of humor has moved in this direction, probably there will be other changes in libidinal interest, such as in pornography or sexual activity. Also, curiosity is distinct from comprehension.

As I previously recounted. Invited to join a meeting of Mensa as a visitor, I was astonished by the absolutely vile dirty and ethnic jokes these geniuses told at their gathering, vying to top one another, with no one taking the least offense, or even palpably reacting. Perhaps the ability to keep a mental distance is a trait of high intelligence, or of people who valorize intellect. The ability to distance oneself from obscene material enough to discuss it, can be assessed as a strength like clinical distance, *or*, as a possible autistic tendency that smart or methodical folks can exhibit.

In evaluating, note and respect religious or cultural taboos that can forbid expression or admission of erotic interest, but not remove it.

The sitcom level of 3-4 can be evaluated by asking about an episode from a favorite recent sitcom, or one that many people saw before the fragmenting advent of cable, such as Lucy (Lucille Ball, in *I Love Lucy*) at the chocolate factory assembly line. Or any *New Yorker* cartoon will do. A more challenging test at this level is asking the person to join in the captioning contest on the last page of every issue of that magazine. Epigrams can also be presented, much in the way we psychiatrists traditionally have proposed proverbs for interpretation, abstraction, and paraphrasing.

The highest level of humor, rated at 4, is the most demanding. It is are emotionally complex humor, and requires a quality of empathy that is universal, having a social awareness that exceeds one's own group. A nuanced subtlety of taste and metaphorical capacity are evident. Examples are not of course limited to my four suggestions, and many more candidates are welcome. Chaucer's *Canterbury Tales* (1387) or Dante's *Divine Comedy* (1368-1370), closely contemporary and both quite funny at times despite their allegory, are less accessible and more difficult to use than asking a patient what is funny about a man so in love with the noble ideal of being a knight that he attacks windmills as giants with long arms (*Don Quixote*, 1608).

Again, it is not any specific examples, but how they exemplify the functional demands of humor at that level. Social satire, such as by Jonathan Swift or by familiar recent comedians such as Richard Pryor, Chris Rock, Dave Chapelle or Eddie Murphy illustrate this level if they rise to universal.

Culture and Language

To repeat from the introductory remarks, in all evaluations one must take education, language and culture into consideration. As I said, psychiatrists often evaluate abstracting and metaphorical capability by asking someone to "interpret" a proverb (or even a figure of speech in a musical lyric). Examples are "Rolling stones gather no moss" which could mean, "if you never settle down you won't accumulate riches" or, alternatively, "if you don't keep moving bad things will grow on you." Any answer that reflects metaphorical intactness should have to do with the human condition and not literally stones or moss. My example of cultural specificity above was that people from Spanish-speaking cultures do better with "The shrimp that falls asleep is carried away by the stream" ("El camerón que se queda dormido es arrastrado por el arroyo"), interpreting it for example as "If you don't pay attention you will be/think like everybody else," or "If a person is not alert they will miss opportunities to move up." No example is universal, but the levels of capacity can be identified in any culture or language. The sense of humor is better valued for its social and interpersonal relevance in its own culture than its ingredient of abstracting ability alone.

Discussion:
Skills of the Humorist and Loci of Humor

The ratings are not of the art or skill necessary to create the humor, but rather the mental capacities that are needed to appreciate it at each level. Nor are the most subtle among us exempt from also enjoying the lower levels of humor: Alexander Romanovitch Luria (1902-1977), the father of neuropsychological assessment, loved puns and jokes, and enjoyed them

sometimes inappropriately at scientific meetings (Homskaya, 2001). Precise neuroanatomic localization is often not possible, because the appreciation of humor at each level would be quite distributed in the brain. Similarly, psychiatry has moved from trying to pin-
point brain regions causing psychiatric disorders to finding linkages of regions forming neural networks or circuits, especially between the prefrontal cortex and the limbic system (Kalin NH, 2019). The specific choices of humor here proposed, from the most complex, subtle, and cognitively and emotionally demanding, to the least demanding, are not set in stone. The spectrum invites additions and emendations at each level, and refinement of neuroanatomic and functional correlations.

Funniness: Humor can be funny at every level, and how funny any example of humor is cannot be superimposed on such a scale. Nor can it be said that the talent and skill required to produce the humor is commensurate with its level. Very low physical comedy or off-color humor may make creative and performance demands. An A-list of the most talented names in comedy vied to deliver their versions of the same notorious dirty (off-color) joke. Needless to say, it was all in the telling or delivery. Penn Jillette and Paul Provenza made their contest into a documentary film, See Appendix, **"The Aristocrats."**

Nature of Laughter: Laughter is a rapidly repetitive and rhythmic contraction of the diaphragm that may be audibly voiced, and that may arise from emotional thoughts or external perceptions that are found funny. It can also arise from being tickled and in meaningless hilarity from certain substances such as nitrous oxide or cannabis. Its neurological situation is the ventromedial prefrontal cortex with involvement of the amygdala and hippocampus, together with the telencephalic and diencephalic respiratory centers. Norman Cousins described laughter as medicinal in effect. Its study is called **gelotology**.

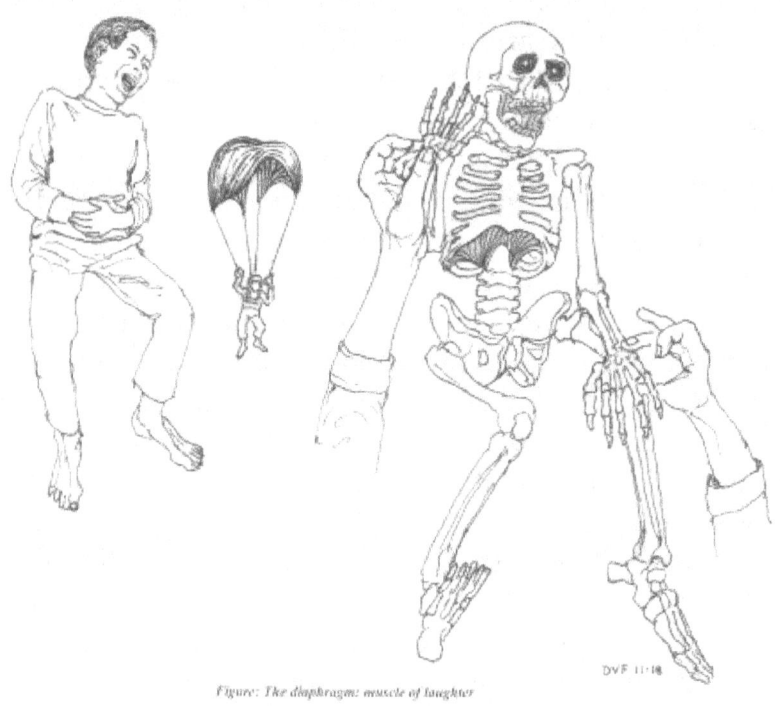

Figure: The diaphragm: muscle of laughter

Figure: The diaphragm: muscle of laughing

The diaphragm is a remarkable muscle that together with the intercostal (rib) muscles produces laughing. It is shaped like a parachute and attached inside the lower ribs where it divides the chest and its organs from the abdomen and its organs. Under both voluntary and reflex control, the versatile diaphragm participates in many familiar bodily functions whose neurology, physiology and interrelatedness is only partly understood. These differ in duration and repetitiveness:

Bearing down (valsalva maneuver, fixing of the diaphragm while holding one's breath), *as in weightlifting, any athletic or physical effort, or forcing defecation.*

Breathing, *in which the diaphragm, as the most important muscle involved, repetitively and automatically expands downward to create a vacuum that draws in air (inhalation), then contracts to exhale. Both actions can be consciously overridden as in speaking, singing and breath holding.*

Yawning *is an automatic deep breath taking involving the diaphragm and intercostals and accompanied by slight tearing. It increases aeration but has a social dimension termed contagious yawning, in which one person yawning induces others (or even one's pets) also to yawn. This requires an empathic sensitivity that may be less in persons with schizophrenic or autistic syndromes.*

Hiccupping (hiccoughing) *is also repetitive diaphragmatic expansion that often occurs by surprise like a tic, and may be audible. It can go on for days with chronic irritation of the phrenic nerve and be profoundly enervating, requiring medication to halt.*

Retching and vomiting (emesis) *require the diaphragm to expand, creating a vacuum that opens the esophagus to help the contracting abdominal and stomach muscles expel stomach contents. On an episode of Discovery Channel's "Dirty Jobs," entitled "Bug Detective"(Episode 139, Season 6, Number 8, first aired November 28, 2010), host Mike Rowe visits Purdue's crime scene investigation Forensic Entomology Research Compound, where they have a farm of pig corpses in different stages of decomposition for calibrating the timing of death by stages in the invasion of insects. The scientists must contend with their rising gorges, and have found that forcing smiling counteracts nausea. This useful pearl of wisdom enlarges the study of facial feedback, and mysteriously unites in an odd way the laughing and retching diaphragm with the facial motion of mirth.*

Coughing (tussis) *occurs when the diaphragm first expands to draw in air, then contracts with the intercostal muscles against a stopped glottis to create pressure, then expel phlegm. Like laughter, coughing is controlled by the medulla oblongata in the brain stem and uses the same muscles. Unsurprisingly, a coughing "fit" often follows a "fit" of laughter. Pathological changes in the brain may impair the protective cough reflex, so that there is benefit from swallowing coaching. Violent coughing occurs in some conditions of spinocerebellar atrophy. In the December/January 2018* Neurology Today, *clean comedian Jim Gaffigan and his wife Jeannie describe her struggle with both problems as a result of a benign spinal cord tumor. Cough can be an odd side effect of ACE (angiotensin-converting enzyme) medications used to lower blood pressure, because* they increase the cough reflex, and their breakdown products, kinins, lodge in the lungs and are slow to clear after the medication is stopped.

Sneezing (sternutation) *is an event in which the diaphragm first draws in air, then vigorously contracts to clear the nasopharynx of mucus. Nasal tickle can cause sneezing but a third of people sneeze with bright light; this and repeatedly sneezing a certain number of times can be inherited. I recently heard a female medical student sneeze five times in five seconds! Sneezing releases endorphins and feels good. It may create a voiced ah-choo. Usually one must be awake to sneeze, but not to cough.*

Sobbing *(as distinguished from silent weeping) resembles laughing, can be combined or alternate with laughing (especially in pathological pseudobulbar lability), and both can be accompanied by tears--as can sneezing and yawning).*

Laughing, *like sobbing, is a rhythmic contraction of the diaphragm several times a second (which may or may not be accompanied by audible heh-heh-heh or ha-ha-ha vocalizations. Humor may be experienced without laughter, and laughter without humor. Unlike sobbing, laughter may result from tickling, but one cannot tickle oneself because it is impossible to surprise one's brain. Tickling is part of bonding with babies. Rodents giggle, too (Panksepp, 2005, Shanor K and Kanwal J, 2011). Provine (2000) has placed laughter in wider social contexts than humor. Laughter facilitates social bonding and can occur in inappropriate situations such as grief or horror. Provine (2000) suggests laughter is more likely in larger social groups in casual situations with lots of face-to-face contact (pp. 209ff).*

Mirthful laughing has been considered beneficial for an individual. Laughter is the best medicine, as the saying goes. Laughter is a major ingredient in social bonding. Adults laugh 15-30 times a day and babies 300 times. Newborns smile and there are many clips on YouTube of babies laughing, often at little things, like a piece of paper being torn. We are 30 times more likely to laugh when we are in a group. But laughter can be stressful, raise the heart rate and blood pressure, and with all its exhalation, cause shortness of breath.

Filippelli and his co-workers(1985) presented 7 subjects with the funniest scenes in a Robert Benigno movie and found the laughing lasted an average of 3.7 +/- 2.25 seconds. There was a drop in the functional residual capacity of the lungs of 1.55 +/- 0.40 liters of air. Facial flushing is common with the exertion.

Cataplexy is an unusual condition caused by laughter and strong emotions, usually in people who have narcolepsy. In a cataplectic attack, which is not to be confused with epilepsy, there is a sudden onset of limpness of the voluntary muscles of the body that hold us up and open our eyes, so the person collapses. This is like the natural muscle paralysis of rapid eye movement sleep that keeps us from enacting our dreaming, but instead, the person is conscious, sometimes with eyes closed and, in a case I witnessed, still holding the abdomen and laughing helplessly on the floor. It is harmless unless the individual is overcome with no safe place to collapse, as when driving. It is distinguished from **catalepsy**, or waxy flexibility in catatonia, associated with mutism and increased muscle tone.

In the 2019 film, Joker, Joachin Phoenix brilliantly conveys the emotional pain of a man who has suffered brain damage, assaults and relationship losses. Most distinctively, he laughs inappropriately at certain times of stress, and the laughing is at times a transition from sobbing. The Joker is a character, not a person, but he has been diagnosed by some reviewers as suffering from **pseudobulbar affect**, which results in excessive and varying emotional outbursts that are not appropriate to situations. Less vehement emotional inappropriateness occurs in schizophrenia. But the Joker's labile laughter is more meaningful. It occurs when he or another person is victimized, seemingly as an overflow of anguish. The film is a tutorial about cruel humor that picks on the weak and different, and at one point manipulates the audience in spite of ourselves into horrified laughter at the plight of a character who is a little person, bringing the lesson painfully home.

On January 5, 2020, Joachin Phoenix received the Golden Globes Award for Best Actor in a Drama for Joker, and on February 9, The Academy Award for Best Actor in a Leading Role.

Humor and the Senses

I have repeatedly noted above that the senses of hearing and/or vision are needed to receive the comic stimulus. Further basic capacities, such as the appreciation of rhythm and tone, or competence in facial recognition and affect appraisal can be added.

But the apprehension of humor is a higher cortical function, and other senses can provide the input. Helen Keller, who had neither vision nor hearing, and was reliant upon touch for language, wrote "The best and most beautiful things in the world cannot be seen or ever touched--they must be felt with the heart" (Keller, 1905).

Itch and **tickling** are dimensions of the sense of touch, as are other tactile and proprioceptive afferent messages (Gopnik, 2016). Could tickling be tactile humor? It arises when light or intimate touch is known or discovered not to be threatening. The same sensation caused by an insect would be creepy formication, causing piloerection (hairs standing on end) and the skin to "crawl." The discrepant or surprise element of jokes is present in tickling, which is why we can't tickle ourselves. Many tactile tricks and illusions seem funny too. Itching (Mochizuki 2014) is carried to the brain via the thalamus and reaches the sensory homunculus and the insula (see immediately below), but at the same time activates the cerebellum, which starts planning how to respond (scratch). The funny bone is a point at the elbow where the ulnar nerve is close to the surface of the skin and, when bumped, tingles.

Figure: Homunculi: the brain's representation of the body

The cortical homunculi were visualized by neurosurgeon Wilder Penfield (Penfield and Boldrey, 1937, Penfield and Rasmussen, 1950) as "grotesque creatures," imagined as a 3-dimensional representation of body parts whose size was proportional to the area of the brain devoted to their sensory or motor function, that is, to the importance our brains give to them. Each of the side surfaces of the brain (for the opposite right and left sides of the body) has a primary motor area and a primary sensory area in front of and in back of the vertical Central (or Rolandic) sulcus (or fissure). This sulcus divides the motoric strip of the frontal lobe and the somatosensory strip of the parietal lobe, and both continue over the top of each hemisphere and down into the Sylvian fissure, where they are called the paracentral gyrus. There is a sensory and a motor homunculus on the left and right side of the brain (for the right and left sides of the body respectively). They lie on the convex surface of the brain with the representations of the head lowest, the waist and buttocks highest, and the legs tucked down into the Sylvian fissure on the paracentral gyrus, and they differ slightly according to anatomical sex. They are inherently funny because, like caricatures, they are incongruous with our images of ourselves. For example, the lips and tongue are enlarged, and the hands are huge at the ends of pipestem arms. There are no genitals on Penfield's electrostimulatory mappings. A statue was fashioned by Sharon Price Jones. She added male genitals in proportion to the small body of the homunculus and much smaller than its huge hands. I found online a statue (sculptor uncertain) that revises that original sensory homunculus by depicting the penis more in proportion to the importance we give it, in other words, huge. Most men and women would agree, in principle, with this penile emphasis in men's minds (and clitoral in women's). This is funny, much as were the phalluses flopping around on the priapic characters in Greek and Roman comedy. But it would seem to be a mystery, where the missing phallic importance lies anatomically. Penfield mapped it below the foot on the paracentral gyrus deep down in the Sylvian fissure that runs from front to back, dividing the left and right hemispheres of the brain. Oddly, it is small. A more recent review of the cortical sensory representation of the genitalia of men and women (Cazala et al. 2015) acknowledged the location remains poorly known, but concluded that there are two distinct areas for genital sensations in the primary somatosensory cortex, one tucked away on the paracentral gyrus on the medial surface and one on the lateral surface. Also, the secondary somatosensory cortex and the posterior insula--an area of cortex one must retract open the lateral fissure to uncover--represent the all-important affective and pleasurable aspects of genital sensation, including feeling tumescence. The clitoris is not overlooked, as it has been in its medical history, but found to be represented where the penis is, on the medial paracentral lobule (gyrus), according to an fMRI study (Komisaruk, et al., 2011), which added that the nipple with its erotogenic potential was also represented there, as well as on the thoracic region of the somatosensory homunculus.

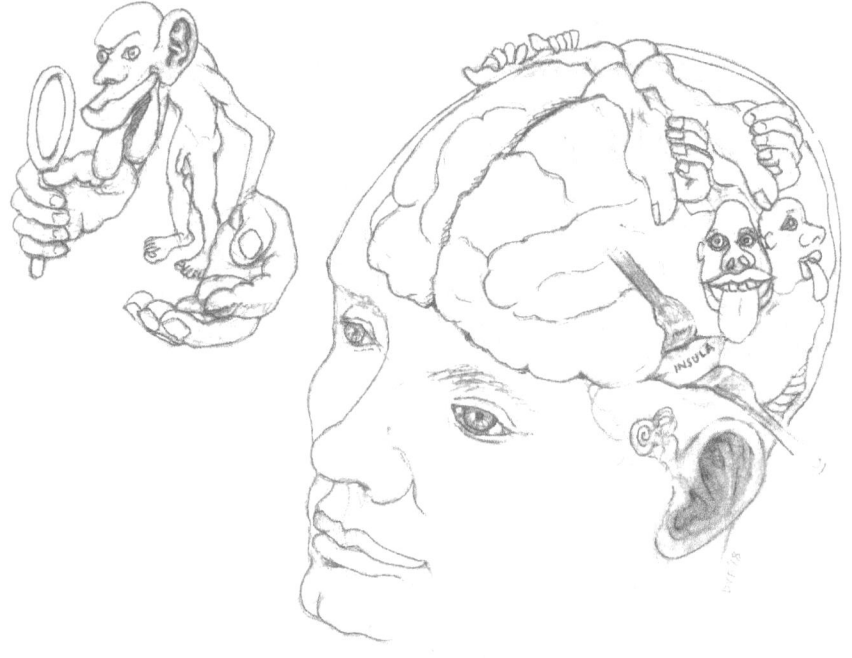

Figure: Homunculi: the brain's representation of the body

Those who might doubt that the linked senses of **smell and taste** could be humorous might try some of the jellybeans manufactured in connection with the Harry Potter films, which surprised the delighted young-at-heart to find in candy not only the flavors Grass, Soap and Rotten Egg, but Dirt, Earthworm, Earwax, Booger and Vomit. Kate McLean has made an Urban Smellscape Aroma Wheel (Lupton E. et al., p. 65) comparable to the classic German Drom Fragrance Wheel. The smell of a fart can be funny if it appears in a socially awkward setting, like the elevator in the 1997 film Liar Liar in which comedian Jim Carrey portrayed a lawyer compelled to tell the truth and confess that he was the culprit.

If there is a sixth sense, we can bank upon it having humor too.

Incongruity Theory

Error detection has been proposed (see Pierce, 2016, referring to Anjan Chatterjee, M.D., a neurologist at U. Penn., and Jessica Black at Boston College) as critical to the getting of a joke. Error detection is needed to appreciate "the incongruity employed to make the funny point." Thus "the short storyline of the joke works to undo the simple assumptions we automatically make at the start," as in Pierce's example, "I went to buy some camouflage trousers the other day but couldn't find any." An "ah-hah" moment is about a surprise element that resolves the incongruity and leads to amusement. The neurology of getting a joke includes a "vast network" of multiple brain regions from the prefrontal cortex to the temporal lobe and the anterior cingulate gyrus, known for its error detection. The authors suggest a core processing area, including the temporo-parietal junction.

Attardo and Raskin (1991) have proposed a general theory of verbal humor. There are many theories of humor, but theirs falls into incongruity theory, upon which many, including Kant, Freud and Bergson relied. Incongruity theory postulates a release of psychic energy wrongly mobilized by false expectations. Attardo (2001, p. 22) explains that making or getting a joke involves tapping into a descendingly determinative hierarchy of "knowledge resources:" (1) script opposition, or the incongruity between 2 alternative hearings or readings of the joke's text, which is central to incongruity theory; (2) logical mechanism, or how the 2 scripts or senses are brought together; (3) situation, or the setting, location, characters, etc.; (4) target, or who is the butt of the joke; (5) narrative strategy or style; (6) and language elements such as words. Attardo and Raskin (1991, p. 71) also show how making substitutions within these knowledge resources can generate any number of different versions of the same light bulb joke (for examples, the butt of the joke can be Californians, psychiatrists or Aggies).

More Neural Correlations

Chan et al. (2015) conducted an fMRI study in Taiwan of 69 healthy volunteer subjects (35 were female, and the average age was 24) to evaluate the basis in the brain of getting jokes. They compared funny with altered unfunny versions of 3 types of verbal jokes in Mandarin. The 3 types were drawn from a classification by Attardo and Raskin (1991) of verbal humor into 5 types of "logical mechanisms," one of their 6 "knowledge resources" (see above, and Appendix). The 3 types chosen were (1) jokes requiring a *inference* bridging a gap not made explicit about consequence, (2) jokes requiring the appreciation of *exaggeration* violating expectations, and (3) jokes requiring *ambiguity* between possible interpretations to be disambiguated. Chan, et al. found the funniness of all 3 types of jokes activated the dorsolateral prefrontal gyrus, "presumably related to cognitive processing" or "script shifting" and the left ventral anterior cingulate gyrus, "presumably related to affective processing" and "a common affective mechanism for joke appreciation and the feeling of amusement for all three joke types." The dorsolateral prefrontal cortex also modulates the amygdala in affective appraisal.

Inference jokes require resolving or bridging incongruities, and inferring others' thinking (theory of mind). The temporo-parietal junction and other medial temporal areas that detect incongruity are needed to "get" these jokes. The temporo-parietal junction is where social perception resides in the brain. Damage at this location impairs attributing intention (Apperly, et al., 2004), required for higher ranked humor.

Exaggeration and *ambiguity* jokes particularly activate the fronto-parietal lobe (bilateral inferior parietal lobe or ventral parietal cortex, and right inferior frontal gyrus). The amygdala and the nucleus accumbens support the dopamine system of emotional reward and may boost the funniness of exaggeration jokes, which employ surprise, distortion and ironic expression.

Summarizing previous literature, Chan, et al. note that the ventrolateral prefrontal gyrus and inferior parietal lobe are thought to attend to rare or novel events, semantic processing, and feeling amused; and the frontal polar cortex, to mentalizing social functions and detecting unexpected exaggeration. These regions are also part of the *mirror circuit* distinguishing oneself from others. Some people who have borderline personality disorders (an unfortunate term) have a *delineation disorder* of the boundary between themselves and others that may impair these empathic types of humor.

Chan et al. in conclusion call for functional connectivity studies between regions, and exploring other logical mechanisms (see Appendix).

Figure: Neuroanatomy of finding funny

The anatomical illustration locates some of the structures mentioned in the perception and appreciation of humor. As in the cover illustration, the propinquity of limbic (emotional brain) structures and the basal ganglia and cerebellum (motor rhythm and timing) is evident. The frontal lobe also contributes to feeling and empathy. Sensory pathways must be intact for funny things to be seen and heard via their channels, and they even do some processing. Abbreviations are AUD C = auditory cortex, CN = caudate nucleus of (motor system), M = mammillary body (of limbic system), A = amygdala (emotions like fear), HC = hippocampus (which initiates memory formation), CA1 = cornu ammonis 1 (subfield of hippocampus implicated in schizophrenia), HT = hypothalamus, connected to P = pituitary (directing hormone release). The thalamus (thalami, actually, as it is paired, and the name meaning a wedding chamber) "marries" many "upper" and "lower" parts of the brain's wiring. New research suggests the central lateral thalamus supports consciousness, which is not to call it the "center," any more than to say there's a focal humorous "funny bone" in the brain (like in your elbow where you can hit your ulnar nerve).

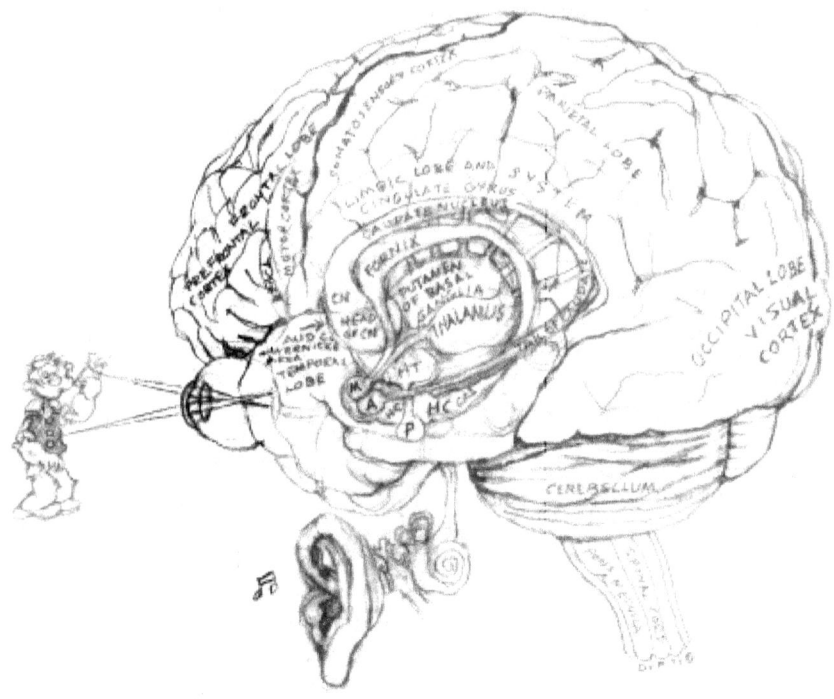

Figure: Neuroanatomy of finding funny

Overview and Conclusion

It is easier to specify categories of logical operations and other cognitive structures involved in types of humor than it is to pinpoint corresponding locations in the neuraxis. Instead, there are broad overlapping regions involved, so the representation of humor is "distributed." We can surmise, with little surprise, that social knowledge for the higher types of humor draws upon prefrontal brain function, and we know
that temporo-parietal regions are involved with language, spatial comparisons, and a host of other basic cognitive operations necessary for comprehension of jokes and the ability to "get" and interrelate the incongruities of a joke. The amygdala adds emotion and the nucleus accumbens pleasure. The march of neuroscience will add granularity to this anatomy; or perhaps more likely, instead of neural pinpoints will identify ever more complex networks that defy our grasp and require computa-

tional mapping, which in turn eventually may further challenge human comprehension to keep up.

Our classification of jokes implies a single dimension of high and low. This is a simplification, like the hierarchy of neuromental capacities for interpersonal interrelatedness (Forrest, 2007). More dimensions can and should eventually be adduced. For example, caricature requires a connectomic network involving not just the amygdala and limbic brain generally, but also a special knowledge of facial, voice and gestural specifics. In places quick and dirty (sometimes literally dirty), the above list of types of humor hopes to offer principles with which to classify what patients find amusing at various stages of maturity, ability, health, aging and neuropathology. More principles and examples are welcome.

Je ne sais quoi - Comedy is more than its content, and that added element is hard to specify or to determine what is needed to appreciate it. Tracy Morgan said of his performances, "It's not about material, it's just being *funny*. Anybody can get material, but you're either funny or you're not" (Cunningham, 2019, p. 38). Jonathan Winters said (Ajaye, pp. 252-3), "Lenny [Bruce] was awfully funny. He was just starting the four-letter word stuff. He thought funny. When a guy is funny, he's funny."

Night fell on the prisoner's first day in jail and he didn't know what to expect. The silence of the lockdown was broken by a voice that called out "37" followed by a roar of laughter. Another voice called out "16" to more laughter and applause. His cellmate said, "we've all been in jail so long we just give each joke a number we all knew." Deciding to try it out, the newbie shouted "28" to a deafening silence. "How come?" he asked. His cellmate replied, "some people can tell 'em."

Emotions of transgression in humor: Much of humor, not just dirty jokes and all manner of offensive humor, is transgressive. If it is based on the violation of social norms, benign or otherwise, as we have noted that thinkers from philosopher Henri Bergson to the cartoon editor of *The New Yorker* have asserted, then the emotions of social transgression are invoked.

And those emotions are the embarrassing feelings of **shame** and **guilt.** Michl et al. (2014) have localized shame and guilt employing fMRI while experimental subjects are imagining shameful and guilt-provoking situations. Both shame and guilt activate the temporal lobe, shame more the anterior cingulate cortex and parahippocampal gyrus, and guilt, more the fusiform gyrus and the middle temporal gyrus. More specifically, shame also activates the medial and inferior frontal gyrus of the frontal lobe, and guilt the amygdala and insula. Shame activates the same frontal and temporal areas in men and women, but guilt activates temporal regions only in
women, and in men additional frontal, occipital and amygdaloid places. Thus these moral/transgressive emotions are located in the frontal, temporal and limbic areas of the brain, and humor can bring them out. Women's stand-up comedy can play with society's traditionally more restrictive expectations of women, and can be all the more transgressive and funny for that. Stand up comedian Louis C.K. frequently employs cringe-worthy, shame-inducing topics.

Empathy: Appreciating how the characters would feel as they are portrayed in humorous situations requires the cognitive capacity for a theory of mind, and empathy. Even when there is a cruel barb to the humor, or the characters who figure in a joke are less than sympathetic, one needs to imagine what they are experiencing. Here is an example:

Elvira had had a long day at the clinic and was on the late train home. As the train slid through the rainy night, she wanted nothing more than to lose herself in her novel.

But no, the guy on the seat next to her took out his cell phone.

"Hello, Lucy, it's Herb! I'm gonna be real late because I had to work late at the office. [pause] No, not with Desirée, she had to leave for a bra fitting. [pause] Just me and the boss. I love only you! Who's your cuddly-wuddly Pooh bear?"

Elvira tried to concentrate on her novel.

"What? Not Carmen, either. She had scheduled a Brazilian bikini wax. It's you I love! Who's your fuzzy-wuzzy panda bear?"

Elvira pretended to read.

"Just the boss and me. [pause] Yes, of *course* my boss is a woman! But Lola is really suffering tonight, she has P.M.S! And who's your big, furry-wurry grizzly bear?"

Elvira could take it no more. She closed her book and leaned over Herb's cell phone to speak:

"Herb, would you PLEASE turn that cell phone off?......And come back to bed!"

Getting this joke requires empathic inferences about the characters. One needs to feel Elvira's increasing exasperation that her quiet personal time is being invaded; that Herb is a rascal, his denials and the cutesy bear images he suggests for himself not only spoiling Elvira's solitude, but causing and failing to remove his wife Lucy's jealousies. More social comprehension is required to realize that Herb knows too much about the intimate bodily matters of his female co-workers, and to sympathize with his wife Lucy's suspicious questioning of him. The punch line relieves the tension one feels mounting in Elvira, who has her revenge by seeming to confirm Lucy's fears about Herb, so that Herb will really catch hell from his wife.

A counterargument: Paul Bloom (2016) has argued that empathy is overrated, that it constricts our vision and entrenches our prejudices because we have limited emotional capacity and are incapable of empathizing with more than a handful of people at one time. I disagree with this cold view. As a corrective to rationality and hand in hand with it, empathy is not only indispensible but integral to the highest functioning of cognitive processes and their basis in brain. The point of this book is that empathy is not limited or simple.

Kindness versus cruelty is a dimension that divides comedians and contributes to the positioning of humor in our rankings, which valorize empathy and kindness and consider a slide into brutishness to be evidence of deterioration of the

sense of humor, possibly because of dementing processes. Although theoreticians, including Freud, have emphasized that humor has targets, comedians differ in endorsing cruelty. Redd Foxx once joked, (Ajaye, p.7), "Hire the handicapped. They're fun to watch." But Jay Leno (Ajaye ,2002, p.
124), contrasting himself with the humor of Andrew Dice Clay, argued that "to be the comedian, you have to be the guy getting hit on the head. Comedy doesn't come from inflicting pain, it comes from getting pain." Ellen DeGeneres (Ajaye, p. 100) said "It's important to be happy." Ironically the ever-sunny Ellen now has a relatively sadistic *Ellen's Game of Games* show (NBC-TV, 2018) in which she pushes a button when contestants miss questions, so the floor of their high platform gives way, dropping them down a tube that rivals Dante's, to the audience's mirth. Ricky Gervais (2020) as a personal rule doesn't make jokes about things people can't help. Exactly!

The computer science department of Northeastern University, trying to "robot-proof" its nerdy majors, has required them to take a course on improvisation, non-technical speaking...and joke telling! (Castellanos 2019), because "empathy, creativity and teamwork help students exercise their competitive advantage over machines," according to the university president Joseph E. Aoun. Let's hope they don't get stuck in the uncanny valley as they get closer to human. I'm kidding--they're students, not robots.

Requires: Empathic response requires intactness of the limbic structures of emotion: the basic neurological substrate of understanding, and reflecting cognitively and emotionally, the actions and movements of others. This involves a lot of the brain, including the putative *mirror neurons* of comprehending and mirroring (imitating) others. In humans, brain activity consistent with that of mirror neurons, which were discovered in monkeys, has been located in the pre-motor cortex, the supplementary motor area, the primary sensory cortex, and the inferior parietal cortex. Structures around the superior temporal sulcus are implicated in social perception (see Acharya S. and

Shukla S, 2012), and are relevant to the cognitive and empathic getting of jokes.

The Brain Is a Time Organ

The brain makes meaning in *spatial* dimensions of representation, including:
(1) developing and rerouting of its wired connectivity;
(2) Hebbian redistribution of emphases in those networks (neurons that fire together wire stronger together);
(3) budding on the dendritic processes and the growth and degeneration of axons;
(4) allocations across synapses of hundreds
of neurotransmitter chemicals, only a fraction of which, in all likelihood, are now known;
(5) a subneuronal network of mitochondria poorly understood;
(6) possible quantum effects as yet even more speculative.

All these ways of representing meaning are *spatial*; that is, actually or hypothetically mappable in three dimensions. Humor dances upon them all in the intangible fourth dimension of *time*, by which the brain becomes the *temporal* dynamic system eloquently suggested by Charles Sherrington in 1942 in a weaving metaphor:

"Swiftly the head mass [brain] becomes an enchanted loom where millions of flashing shuttles weave a dissolving pattern, always a meaningful pattern, though never an abiding one; a shifting pattern of subpatterns" (Sherrington, 1942).

If the innumerable places in the brain were merely connected in a static grid, there would be no learning, thinking or action. It would merely be a sort of pinball machine in which the launched ball of attention bounced around lighting the fixed stanchions. While memory is a bit like this, the brain is far more complicated. Brain activation occurs in a time frame as the **synchrony** of correlated sites, and brain work can be traced (very coarsely) over time by fMRI abetted by optogenetic tagging. EEGs also track shifting brain regions and show a fundamental quality of brain electricity: waves, both background rhythms and its signifying overwriting. Too much or generalized synchrony simplifies waves to become literally a brain storm or seizure. Synchrony is a basic element of all moving life (Strogatz, 2004).

Despite all the mechanisms for the encoding of spatial information, how the brain encodes (puts a time stamp on) memories has remained mysterious. Starting with observations that neural cells can fire in sequences, psychologists like Marc Howard (Howard, et al., 2013) have worked with mathematical physicists like Karthik Shankar (Shankar, et al., 2016) to determine how the brain makes a timeline (see summary by Cepelewicz, 2019). This involves the complex math of reverse (Laplace) transforms--a mathematical reverse engineering--that demonstrates that the time stamping of episodic (declarative) memory is real, at least for millions of seconds. Thus there is a phase precession of the theta (EEG) rhythm of neurons in the hippocampus and ventral striatum. Shankar et al (2016, p. 2615) explain that "the hypothesis assumes that time and place cells observed in the hippocampus represent time or position as a result of a 2-layer [neural network] architecture that encodes and inverts the Laplace transform of external output." Rat work (by Tsao, discussed in Cepelowicz, (2019) may even explain why the perception of time is so elastic.

It is wondrous to contemplate how even the timing of a joke relies upon a temporal underpinning of neural network mechanisms of such complexity.

As suggested by the EEG, and the precession of theta sync of nerve cells just described, the hallmark of brain activity is that is **rhythmic**. Some examples of how we "got rhythm" include many everyday repetitive muscular functions with frequency or periodicity. Many have to do with ejection or riddance from the body:

Rhythmic, repeating bodily movements of less than one second periodicity include: flagellation (of sperm), ciliation (of hair cells), heartbeat, tremor, shudder, shiver, tremble, hiccough, cough, laugh, sneeze, yawn, and eyeblink. Rhythmicities with periodicities equal to or more than 1 second include: ejaculation, climax, breathing, peristalsis, defecation, emesis, parturition and walking or swimming.

All EEG rhythms have a <1 sec periodicity. But the rhythmic movements of the body often have longer periods, and perhaps can be explained as emergent assemblages or harmonics of brain waves (linked oscillations). However they are composed, brain generators produce rhythmic discharges that effect movements at varying frequencies. **Tremor** results from an asynchrony of the balance between flexor and extensor muscles. Perhaps a steady limb is one in which the rhythms of the sets of opposing muscles are synchronized in perfect cancellation, as in noise cancellation. Dr. Sheng Kuo (personal communication, March 21, 2019) has been able to bypass the inferior olivary cerebellar input into a cerebellar Purkinji neuron of a mouse, and to stimulate tremors at frequencies he chooses. This demonstrates that the cerebellum alone can create the synchrony of a tremor and, perhaps analogously, so many other coordinated activities of brain and mind. Strogatz (2004), an applied mathematician, has explained in a landmark book how physical and biological systems can self-organize into synchrony. I think the question in tremor is how flexor and extensor muscles can desynchronize--or how each can *synchronize* contractions *out of phase* with the other in regular alternation. The aberration seems even more amazing.

Widge and Miller (2019) at MIT hypothesize purposes for different EEG brain rhythm oscillations. Bottom-up processing of incoming information generates gamma (>30 Hz) oscillations through the cortex. Top-down focus of attention generates alpha (8-15 Hz) or beta (15-30 Hz) that suppress gamma and order thought. Slower theta waves (5-8 Hz) synchronize prefrontal and limbic system activity for self-regulation. Widge and Miller propose that strong gamma with over-attention to bottom-up processing causes attention deficit, while diminished gamma oscillations causes schizophrenia, so information doesn't get in. They propose precisely-timed neurostimulation as an eventual future fix to return brain waves to "orchestrated synchrony."

Brain generators are not well understood. They interact with their target organs, some of which, like the heart, have an inherent rhythmicity even when neurally disconnected. Some of the target organs have innervation that is less direct, peripheral or autonomic.

Figure: Timing in the brain and in humor

In 2017 the Nobel Prize in Physiology or Medicine was awarded jointly to Jeffrey C. Hall, Michael Rosbash and Michael W. Young, who discovered in fruit flies the molecular mechanisms controlling the circadian rhythm. 3 genes are instrumental: "period," which accumulates by night and is degraded by day; "timeless," which can lock the period gene's activity, and "doubletime," which controls the oscillation to fit a 24 hour cycle. This is also the basis of our cycle around the hours of the day.

The **cerebellum** coordinates the timing of many bodily movements, and its impairment results in clumsiness, poor targeting (past pointing) and trouble with rapid successive movements, called dysdiadochokinesis. The full extent of cerebellar coordination involves mental as well as motor activity, and was explored in collaboration with leading neuroscientists by Fred Levin (2009). Relying on Masao Ito's controller-regulator of the brain, Levin argued for cerebellar influence upon emotion in the coordination of implicit memory (knowing how) and explicit memory (knowing what). Correspondingly, Schmahmann's syndrome (cerebellar cognitive affective syndrome, or CCAS) (Hoche et al., 2018) from cerebellar impairment features problems with

executive functions such as working memory, mental flexibility, abstract reasoning, semantic fluency and attentional and emotional control, without affecting the Mini-Mental State Exam (MMSE) or the Montreal Cognitive Assessment (MCoA) scores. But these cerebellar executive impairments should prove relevant to the appreciation of humor and its timing.

THE LAUGHING BRAIN

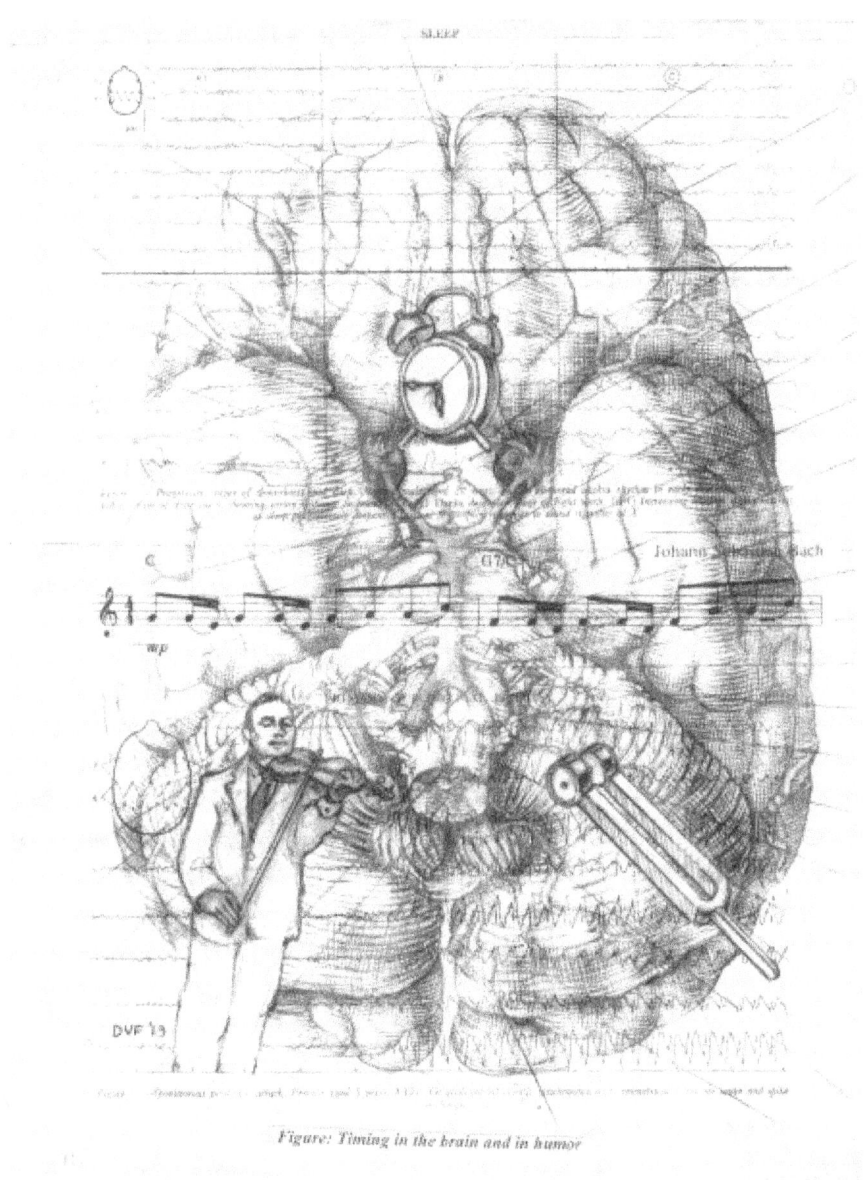

Figure: Timing in the brain and in humor

Comedic timing - *Much humor depends for its effect on timing, especially in dialogue, repartee and joke telling, in which the ten-*

sion of the set up builds to a surprise. Comedians rely on it and some comedians are notable for it, such as Jack Benny, who manipulated rising expectation with a simply timed "Well." He did routines with Mel Blanc such as "si sew Sue" and "What's in a Name" (1957), in which Blanc's supposed spittle-producing name Gropff led Blanc to dry his face every time Benny said it. Benny milked delays with his violin much as Victor Borge did with his piano. Borge also invented humorous punctuation signs for music in 1955, which he later performed faultlessly with a (customarily) unrehearsed but ever graceful Dean Martin.

Franklin Ajaye (2002) collected interviews from stand-up comedians (like himself), and considered that timing enters into comedy at 2 points: delivering the punch line and allowing an interval between jokes after the audience laughs. "Good pauses" are essential (pp. 13-15). Ajaye (p.14) added, "Jack Benny, that late, great master of timing and space, once said, 'if I take the time to wait to tell them, those silences are as strong as the words.'" Rushing to the next joke (before at least 2 seconds) "puts brakes on" laughter and may obscure subtler "afterthought" lines. "Let the laughter run its natural course. Then, before it drops into total silence, start the next routine. This way you build an almost **musical rhythm** [emphasis mine] that has its own natural ebbs and flows" (Ajaye himself, p. 14). A pause before delivering the punchline "lights the fuse" to the joke (Ajaye, p. 20). Roseanne (Ajaye, p. 188) confessed she "stole timing off" W.C. Fields, thereby underscoring that time is a real, even proprietary element in humor. Jerry Seinfeld (Ajaye p.199) noted that beginning comedians don't "know that you're talking too fast or that you're talking in a rote fashion instead of in the present moment."

Cerebral palsy and other developmental delays may lead to abnormal timing of speech. Parkinsonian patients, whose basal ganglia are undersupplied with dopamine from the substantia nigra (which releases it in timed pulses) develop slowing of their moving (bradykinesia) and thinking (bradyphrenia). They may also have uncontrollable acceleration of their footsteps (festination) and speech (tachyphemia) with involuntary repetition of syllables (palilalia).

Joseph Jaffe et al. (2002), working with Beatrice Beebe, found that the coordination of interpersonal timing (CIT) of vocalizations between mothers and their infants at 4 months predicted their social and cognitive development at 12 months. Jaffe and his collaborators employed early computers in the 1960s (I remember their punch cards when I was on a research elective supervised by Jaffe in 1961), to study the mathematically lawful alternation and coordination of sounds by mother and infant, independent of content. This led to understanding that infants are active in dialogue and their cognitive development is inextricable from their social development. This would resemble bird song, with both congenital components and a tutoring of the offspring. The CIT techniques could be applied to adult conversational exchanges and no doubt to the humor of Benny and Blanc. In point of fact, Blanc's repeatedly sudden reply of "si" (yes), delivered with his gaze fixed on Benny, was a critical contribution of timing to the humor of the routine.

Thus timing is essential to rapport development and humor. The timing of humor is crucial: telegraphing or overly delaying a punch line kills a joke, and rapport both promotes humor and is promoted by humor. Humor is one of the best means of bridging a social or cultural or social gap, and laughing together can seal rapport in a relationship.

Robots Crack but Don't Get Jokes

Since the early 1990's artificial intelligence has been able to crack a joke (Marshall A, 2015). A pair of apparently-not-so-dour Scottish computer scientists (Binsted and Ritchie, 1994) created a program that produced punning humor by such devices as syllable substitution, for example, "What do near-sighted ghosts wear? Spooktacles"; and word substitution, for example, "How do you make gold soup? Put 24 carrots in it"; or "What do you call a good-looking taxi? A handsome cab" (Robot jokes aren't always that funny). AI also created metathesis (spoonerisms) such as "What's the difference between a short witch and a fleeing deer? One's a stunted hag and the other a hunted stag"; and inserted short sound-alike words into longer terms and phrases, for example, "What do you give a nervous elephant? A *trunk*quilizer." These rank low on our rating scale, and resemble children's humor, as described above. Made by a computer, these puns were *selected by humans* who knew *that* they were funny and *why*.

On the other hand, robots may differ from humans by their inability to *get* humor (Associated Press, April 2019). Computational linguist Kiki Hempleman at Texas A & M says it's because they miss context. Even puns can require huge amounts of background to know *why* they are funny.

Allison Bishop at Columbia points out that a computer looks for patterns but humor hovers close to a pattern and then veers off "to skate the edge of being cohesive enough and surprising enough." Noam Sloni, who wrote an Israeli version of *Saturday Night Live,* says comedy relies on context and timing. I imagine Jack Benny would be impossible for a robot to get, even from the front row. Hempleman fears teaching robots humor may risk them doing dangerous things, such as *literally* killing if it seemed funny to them. She jokes robots may exceed us, but not because they are getting smarter.

Take-home lessons may result from these computer studies. One is a systematic specification of the mechanisms of humor production and comprehension. The other is that getting humor is a very human thing and, as this essay has been contemplating, a measure of an intact human mind and brain. The study of computational humor models may one day contribute to studies of mind in health and disease.

A brief orientation to dementing disorders

A caution: The following descriptions of relevant neuropsychiatric disorders, although written for both health professionals and general audiences, elaborate some of the most severe symptoms and impaired processes that can affect brain and mind. Reading about them may be upsetting to some, especially if they or their loved ones now have some impairments that could be perceived as residing along the same spectrum of disability. If such discomfort is anticipated, some readers may prefer to consider the ranking of humor as enough, and move on to the Appendix.

Dementia is loss of memory, that is the retention and recollection of what has been perceived, registered and learned, as well as loss of other faculties such as executive planning, ordering, sequencing, and carrying out one's affairs. It often arises from **internal** processes. Certain dementing degenerative diseases also interfere with the comprehension of humor, especially if they affect such brain functions as abstraction, comparison, working memory, shifting of one mental set to another (which occurs with punch lines), salience, and empathy. A preserved knowledge of social norms is needed with which to compare violations of expectation, a recognized basis for humor. Often long term or old memories are remembered while short term memory of recent events are not. Vocabulary is a capacity that is usually well-preserved in normal older people (who love *Wheel of Fortune*) along with long-ago acquired explicit or declarative factual knowledge (*Jeopardy*). But memory for names may be affected, mildly in middle age forgetting, and profoundly in dementias affecting the cortex of grey matter. Dementias affecting the deeper white matter affect thought processing speed. Implicit know-how for familiar actions such as bicycle riding tends to stay longer. Knowing a visitor is a familiar or even loved person may persist while forgetting who the person is. Many other functions may be affected, some that people might not know they possessed, or may not miss, such as copying geometric figures or substituting symbols.

Dementia must be distinguished from **delirium**, or being unable to pay enough attention to perceive, focus on, understand, or record information from the world. Memories are not retrieved because they have not been laid down in the first place. Delirium lowers the sensorium, which is the level of consciousness and awareness. We all experience a healthy version of it when we are very sleepy and cannot read further or pay attention any longer. I have fallen asleep typing this manuscript and roused to find my finger resting on a key that had filled much of the rest of the page with the same letter.

Delirium commonly results from **external** causes. Older patients who have been taking certain medications for years or decades without trouble may slip into delirium when their systems that metabolize and eliminate the medications slow down, so that the same previously helpful intake is too much, and the medications or their metabolic products build up, fogging consciousness. Adjusting the dosage downward reverses the delirium. Delirium tends to come on rapidly, and dementia more gradually. There are chronic deliria, however, such as the mild befogging of shift workers who cannot fully adjust their sleep rhythms and are never fully awake. In the confused states of delirium, the sense of humor may not be lost as long as one can still focus on the joke.

Reversible dementias with a clear consciousness may also occur from such imbalances as low thyroid function and Vitamin B12 deficiency, or the pseudodementia of depression. Emil Kraepelin's name for schizophrenia was *dementia praecox,* or early de
mentia, and in recent years the cognitive problems that accompany the syndrome have again received the attention Kraepelin gave them (Strauss et al. 2018, Kendler 2018). Schizophrenic people have trouble with the comparisons and metaphors in humor, and their stream of thought can become derailed by words with multiple meanings. One schizophrenic patient, speaking of the exhaust of a car, slipped into talking about being exhausted.

Alzheimer's Disease. Richard Mayeux, M.D., addressing Columbia's Neurology Department, of which he is Chairman, at Grand Rounds of November 16, 2018, described the Alzheimer Disease Sequencing Project, which is in search of predisposing genes present across large populations, such as the apoprotein E gene and protein-disrupting variants of the ABCA7 gene. He cited the worldwide incidence of Alzheimer's as 46.8 million people in 2015, projected to be 74.7 million by 2030 and 131.5

by 2050. He continued that in the past, we have spoken of Alzheimer's as a single disease, but pathological studies of those who die of it show only 20-30% have the previously designated hallmark features of amyloid plaques and neurofibrillary tangles. 30% have Lewy bodies, which are present in greater numbers in Lewy Body Dementia (LBD). These are round inclusions in the cytoplasm of neurons that are made up of alpha-synuclein protein. And as many as 50-70% have cerebrovascular lesions (blood vessel clogging) that could have impeded blood supply to the brain (hypoperfusion).

On magnetic resonance imaging (MRI) of Alzheimer patients, the affected areas of the cerebral cortex appear atrophic (shrunken), the gyri withered, with the result that the fissures and sulci that separate them are deeper, and the ventricles (in the center of the cerebrum, which contain cerebrospinal fluid) are enlarged. To add to the Alzheimer's puzzle, Dr, Mayeux continued, MRIs of healthy (asymptomatic) control subjects have revealed that 50-60% have white matter disease, 1/3 have lacunae (small infarction scars), and 10% wedge-like (larger) infarcts. Dr. Mayeux said many of these people would later become demented. At one time vascular dementia was thought more distinct from senile dementia of the Alzheimer type, but now the overlap is acknowledged to be usual. Diagnosis and the search for treatments is complicated by frequently mixed neuropathologic pathology with non-Alzheimer tauopathies and proteinopathies, including a mimicking disorder called LATE (Limbic-predominant Age-related TDP-43 Encephalopathy) (Nelson, et al. 2019; Bowser 2019).

Researchers are frustrated by the ineffectiveness of new therapies that reduce amyloid and the low effectiveness of the drugs approved decades ago. They struggle to assemble Alzheimer's features into a coherent story, including new findings that common viruses like herpes may initiate an immune component. As Belluck (2018) quotes neuroscientist Rudolph Tanzi, "we spent too long thinking about amyloid as plumbing--how much do you produce, how much do you clear. Then we came along and were saying infection is actually driving the amyloid hypothesis. Amyloid's the match, the tangles are a brush fire being spread as they kill neurons, and the virus is lighting the match."

People with **Down syndrome** from trisomy (having an extra copy) of chromosome 21, who once died of cardiac causes by the age of 10, are now living to 65, but 80% have Alzheimer's (Rafil et al., 2018). Humor may be well preserved; as it typically also is in **Huntington's disease**, which is inherited dominantly, and produces both choreic movements and dementia.

A particular type of dementia that impairs one's comprehension and emotional response to humor is **frontotemporal dementia (FTD)**. At one time dementias that were localized to certain lobes were called Pick's disease and the mnemonic was "Pick's picks the lobe." FTD is an umbrella term that includes a behavioral variant (bvFTD). a semantic variant of primary progressive aphasia (svPPA) and a nonfluent/agrammatic variant (nfvPPA). There is also a logopenic ("word-lacking") variant that often has more general Alzheimer findings on autopsy, and a small number of FTD/MND with motor neuron disease (ALS or amyotrophic lateral sclerosis). Neurologists tend to split rather than lump.

Parkinson's disease (PD) primarily originates with loss of dopamine-making cells in the substantia nigra of the midbrain, which is located in the brain stem below the cerebral cortex. Parkinson's responds dramatically to medications that restore dopamine. Its symptoms, which progress slowly over decades, are shaking (of the hands or other parts of the body) at rest, slow and stiff movement, loss of facial expressiveness and voice loudness, cramped handwriting that gets smaller as they write, poorer sense of smell, feeling faint, more sweating and saliva, and trouble swallowing. The movement symptoms often develop asymmetrically, more on one side of the body, which is unusual in degenerative disorders. Symptoms that overlap with primarily psychiatric conditions include a flat or unhappy face, stooped or contracted posture, trouble sleeping. dizziness, constipation, lowered sex drive, and anxiety or depression. Dementia is not prominent, but may occur much later. Poorer spatial perception may accompany the trouble moving, and may lead to overestimating the difficulty of accomplishing actions, or resisting any changes.

Parkinson plus conditions affect additional areas of the brain and are more troubling. They include:

Progressive supranuclear palsy (PSP);

Multiple system atrophy (MSA, or Shy-Drager syndrome);

Corticobasal degeneration;

Diffuse Lewy Body disease.

Progressive supranuclear palsy (PSP) affects the brain nuclei that control gazing up and down, and the pursuit (following) by the gaze. When tracking a moving object, it is jerky or difficult to initiate. Blinking diminishes and the eyes may be dry. The patients tend to fall backwards whereas Parkinson patients tend to fall forwards, often when the PD patient impulsively lunges toward a chair they are aiming for. PSP patients have such Parkinson symptoms as slow gait with freezing (being stuck in place), soft, slow speech and trouble swallowing, but only 10% shake versus 70% of Parkinson patients. The patients are usually older, over 60. PSP progresses more rapidly than typical Parkinson's and dopamine helps only at first. The MRI shows shrinkage at the top of the brainstem (hummingbird sign). PSP patients may be less demented but have difficulty with executive function. Weakness of downward (or upward) eye movements may occur, with shuffling, imbalance, falls, personality changes, speech slurring with the softness of voice and loss of fluency (choked quality), dystonia, impulsivity, impaired abstract thought, labile (pseudobulbar) affect, and depression. Executive impairment affects humor.

Multiple system atrophy (MSA) is a rare and non-familial variant that also progresses faster than typical Parkinsonism. In addition to typical Parkinson movement difficulties they have cerebellar signs of poor coordination, clumsiness, imbalance and staggering, autonomic system issues such as urgency and frequency of urination with incomplete emptying, constipation, impaired potency, difficulty swallowing, and neck and shoulder pain in a coat hanger distribution from postural low blood pressure. Typically they sleep poorly and have snoring and noisy breathing when awake. With all these problems they may be anxious, depressed or overwhelmed. But despite their incapacitation by so many symptoms arising in the brain stem and affecting activities of daily living, they may retain their empathy and sense of humor. This is likely because of the relative sparing of frontal cortical areas. A hot cross bun sign appears on the (axial) MRI looking down on the pons, reflecting pontocerebellar atrophy). MSA is a rare and non-familial disorder which may also have impaired speech fluency, swallowing, eating and breathing, excessive daytime sleepiness, dystonia, and myoclonus. Tremor is less than in Parkinson's, but occurs when the limb is in use rather than at rest. Although rapidly progressing, of the 3 synucleinopathies, MSA is the most likely to lead to great disability with preserved cognition and sense of humor. There are two types, one more associated with cerebellar pathology, ataxia and anxiety; and one more with parkinsonism, associated with depression and problems with executive function, which is easily evaluated (Dubois, 2000). Whereas dementia was once considered an exclusion criterion for MSA, as defined in the American Psychiatric Association's DSM-5 classification, this executive dysfunction, if present, could impair the sense of humor.

Corticobasal syndrome is rare but occurs in the prime of life, even in the 40s. The speech is slurred, and there is trouble swallowing. Stiffness, tremor and apraxic inability to know how to use a hand may occur on one side only. This last produces the odd symptom of *alien hand*, in which a person feels a limb is not part of the body and uncontrollable. It is sometimes called "Dr. Strangelove syndrome," a disability portrayed for darkly comic effect in the 1964 Kubrick film, in which the German rocket scientist cannot restrain his arm from levitating to make a Nazi salute. For example, the patient may lose the ability to use a TV controller. Difficulty with calculation (acalculia) occurs; also dystonia (painful, wry twisting of a limb); dementia with speech problems (stuttering, slurring); some imbalance, asymmetric clumsiness of legs or arms, apraxia, myoclonus and motor freezing.

Lewy Body Dementia (DLB) is an umbrella term for disorders beginning with dementia, movement disorders or psychiatric symptoms. Eventually there can be spreading so that all three symptom categories are present, but in varying degrees, and subtypes have been described based on the distribution of these intranuclear inclusions, with corresponding symptoms. When the frontal lobes are relatively spared, so may be a relatable sense of humor which, while not a completely saving grace in a dementia picture, can be a comfort to loved ones. At autopsy the brain may appear grossly normal. Dementia with Lewy bodies is the third most common dementia after Alzheimer's and vascular dementia. Lewy body nuclear inclusions occur in other disorders like Alzheimer's and Parkinson's diseases, but not in such number, or so generally distributed through the cortex. DLB is characterized by visual hallucinations, often of children or animals or, in one case, brightly-colored insects in a marching band along the baseboard of the room. Often the patient doesn't mind the hallucinations, or finds them pleasant or funny, and I have seen patients with well-preserved humor and cheeriness. Much depends on the extent and distribution of the Lewy bodies. The dementia accompanies or precedes the Parkinsonian motor symptoms rather than the reverse, but there is tremor, stiffness and rapid fluctuations in alertness and attention span, imbalance and falls. There may be confusion, difficulty with familiar faces or objects, spatial awareness, carrying out routine tasks, and word finding. REM behavior disorder (RBD) occurs, a sleep disturbance of physically enacted dreams. DLB responds poorly to first generation antipsychotic medications, but quetiapine (second generation, atypical) can help.

Other neurological disorders that could affect the sense of humor include:

Creutzfeldt-Jakob disease, a rapidly progressing prion disease (85% sporadic, 10-15% hereditary and <1% acquired by ingestion or implantation of affected tissue). George Balanchine, the great choreographer of the New York City Ballet, died of it. In *kuru*, as this contagious prion disease is called in Guam, inappropriate meaningless hilarity may occur as a pathological sign in the early stages (Provine, 2000, p. 155). It is related to mad cow disease (BSE).

Chronic traumatic encephalopathy (CTE/dementia pugilistica) is very much currently in the news because of NFL cases and a new reluctance of parents to permit their children to play tackle football. Since the classic description by Corsellis et al. (1978), there have been questions about attributable symptoms and distinction from or synergy with Alzheimer's (Mayeux, et al., 1995) or military blast CTE.

Schizophrenia is a syndrome of the "positive symptoms" of delusional thinking, auditory rather than visual hallucinations, and a mismatch between feeling and thinking; and also the "negative symptoms" of flattened emotionality, apathy, and lack of will power and motivation. I am including it with the dementias in accord with Emil Kraepelin (1896), who described it as *dementia praecox*, or early dementia, contrasting it with manic depressive illness characterized by major mood swings. Many patients have an overlap syndrome called schizoaffective, with both mood swings and a residual thought disorder. We now know schizophrenia has a relative hypofrontality (Ingvar, et al. 1974, Ziauddeen et al, 2010))--less blood flow in the front of the brain--which correlates with difficulty with logical switching. abstract metaphors and humor. There are language difficulties (Forrest 1976) that include derailing at vulnerable points of language in which a word has multiple meanings (polysemy) or sounds like another (homophony). This is not punning, which requires some language mastery, but rather an enslavement to accidents inherent in language. For example, one schizophrenic patient became derailed from speaking of lawyers to liars. Metaphorical incapacity, or trouble understanding figures of speech and getting stuck on the literal or concrete referents of a metaphorical comparison, creates problems for schizophrenic persons, and also for those on the autistic spectrum with whom they share some idiosyncrasies. Often it is the everyday emotional significances of metaphors and idioms that are troublesome in both cases, and difficulty with the humor that pertains.

Incipient or pre-syndromal schizophrenia is often an activated state, the brain on fire, in which there is a breakdown of mental barriers, such that the person is flooded with perceptions, searching for signposts, and desperate to make sense of things. One such patient, when I asked him what was meant by the saying, "Two heads are better than one," instantly replied, "With two heads you can think twice." Corresponding to this phenomenological description, there is overactivity in the front part (CA1) of the hippocampus, leading to stimulatory dopamine release (Small SA, et al, 2011, Lieberman JA, Small SA, Garhgis RR, 2019).

Contagious humor, like contagious yawning, requires empathic sensitivity, and is likely to be lessened in schizophrenia and autistic syndromes.

The dementias may also be contrasted by the **type of pathological protein that accumulates** in the brain and whether primarily motor or mental (Table):

Table: Pathological types classified two ways:

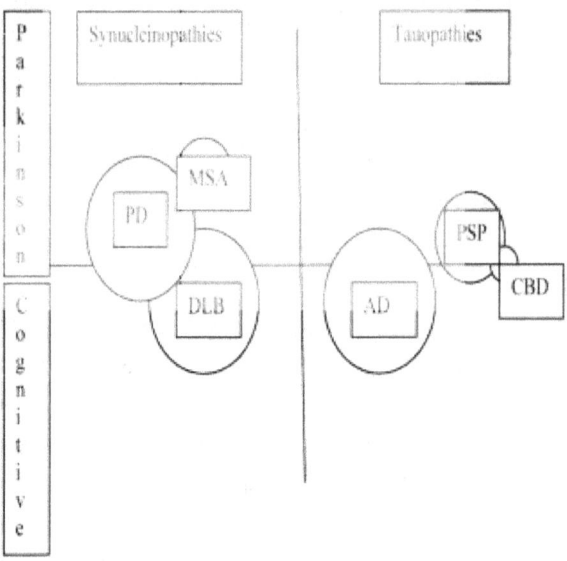

(1) The **alpha-synucleinopathies** include:
    Parkinson's Disease (PD), primarily from degeneration of the substantia nigra
    Lewy Body Dementia (LBD)
    Multiple System Atrophy (MSA
(2) The **tauopathies** include:
    Alzheimer's Disease (AD), which can have a frontal variant
    Chronic Traumatic Encephalopathy (CTE), as from athletes' concussions
    Corticobasal Degeneration (CBDG
    Frontotemporal Lobar Degeneration (FTD)
    Behavioral Variant FTD
    Pick's Disease (an older eponym for frontal lobe degeneration)
    Progressive Supranuclear Palsy (PSP).

Dementias differentiated by frontal lobe function:

The location of pathological changes affects specific faculties needed for humor. The frontal lobes are of special interest because many faculties are found there: conceptualization and abstract reasoning, mental flexibility (the ability to switch between mental sets, evaluated in the Stroop Test and Wisconsin Card Sort), motor programming and executive control of action, resistance to interference, self-regulation, inhibitory control and environmental autonomy. Dubois et al. (2000) introduced a brief battery of 6 subtests to evaluate each of these functions of the frontal lobe. Abstract reasoning is tested by abstract similarities between 2 objects such as an apple and a banana (that they are fruits, not a concrete or perceptual attribute like color). Mental fluency is tested by saying as many words as one can beginning with a given letter in 1 minute. Motor programming is evaluated by Luria's fist-palm-edge test. Interference sensitivity is tested by tapping once when the examiner taps twice, that is, not echoing. Inhibitory control is *not* tapping when the examiner does. Environmental autonomy requires not taking the examiners' proffered hand (prehension) after being asked not to. Another test of frontal (executive) function (as well as parietal lobe visuospatial function) is drawing a clock with a specified time on its face.

Edward Huey (2019), a leading clinical researcher of frontal lobe dementia, also emphasized the importance of the frontal lobe in emotion, postulated upon its connection with the amygdala (which he thinks may be overemphasized as the center of emotion, or even the location of the freudian id!). In Huey's clinical experience, which he illustrated with video clips, FTD patients do not care or suffer anxiety as much when discussing their condition as do other patients with dementias. Huey added that when FTD patients are inconsiderate or even violent, they tend to act without much passion.

This insouciance can be related to a deficit of empathy, needed for the appreciation of higher-ranked humor.

A **preserved sense of humor** in itself suggests intactness of frontal lobe function, and is arguably **a more socially rele-**

vant faculty than other faculties tested above. It is crucial to distinguish sense of humor (comprehension) from hilarity (and lability of moods), which may occur without the ability to get (understand) the humor; and to assess how high on the hierarchy the empathic understanding of humor reaches. Inappropriate emotion may occur in schizophrenia. Extreme mood lability may be **pseudobulbar affect**. This occurs in FTD and may include false laughter, and "emotional incontinence," which is to say, sudden, intense, uncontrollable episodes of crying and/or laughing. It is caused by neurological disease or injury.

Cases contrasted regarding preservation of empathy and sense of humor:

Case 1. Senior forgetting without loss of sense of humor:

A retired and widowed businesswoman in her late seventies developed fears of losing memory. Her neurologist, who had been treating her for neuropathy and joint pains with prednisone, now reduced to 20 mg. a day, and gabapentin, ordered an MRI which was unremarkable. Ahead of neuropsychological testing, she returned to me for a consultation--as I had previously prescribed citalopram for depressive symptoms--now complaining of anxiety, which caused forgetfulness. When anxious, she could not call up words easily in a foreign language conversation course. I determined from her ability to read novels and non-fiction books in 2 languages and other evidence that she was not too seriously impaired, but most convincing of her intactness was the preservation of her subtle sense of humor. This was evident in her telling me how much she had laughed at *Love and Friendship,* a 2016 film adaptation of a Jane Austen story, in which women manipulate men. She also understood and recalled the plot of the film despite having missed the formal *dramatis personae* at the beginning of the film. And she empathically noticed I was moving stiffly because my back hurt. But 3 years later her poorer memory led to assisted living.

Sometimes synucleinopathies and tauopathies overlap in various topistic ways.

Case 2. Dual proteinopathies of **MSA and Alzheimer's** with relative preservation of cognition and humor:

A teacher in her late seventies came to autopsy after succumbing to motor and autonomic features of **multiple system atrophy (MSA)** with dual protein accumulation. She had Parkinson's and Alzheimer's features, but retained enormous cognitive reserve. Even when she became wheelchair bound and incontinent, developed severe respiratory stridor, and required total assistance with her activities of daily living, her cognitive ability was unusually preserved. Most of the degeneration was posterior, with basal ganglia, limbic and olivopontine degeneration. Orotactile and parageusic hallucinations (as if a film on her teeth and abnormal taste) were attributed to involvement of the nucleus solitarius. Eventually she developed some inappropriately labile (pseudobulbar) hilarity, but until late in the course was able to enjoy humor with her loving and supportive family, probably because of relatively less frontal cortical involvement, typical of MSA.

There are **variants of MSA** that are more parkinsonian, affecting executive function and associated more with depression, or cerebellar, with more ataxia and anxiety; but when there is less frontal lobe involvement there is more likelihood of retention of a sense of humor in this otherwise very disabling disease.

Case 3. Frontotemporal dementia with nonfluent aphasia and loss of sense of humor:

A retired interior designer in his middle seventies began 4-5 years ago to struggle "to spit out words," more in English than his native Spanish, according to his wife who said he also "became moody, aggressive and would slam things." His speech became telegraphic; instead of "It is a nice day," he would just say "day'" or "nice." He stopped finding things funny, but at times laughed inappropriately. Noticeably ashamed of his disability, he stayed in his room, but came down punctually to make himself meals, alternately a salad or pasta. His wife said the last thing he laughed at was when she yelled at their dog. Asked what made him happy, he tried to speak, but instead pointed to his wife seated next to him and smiled proudly. Imaging showed atrophy at the top of his cerebrum, midbrain and cerebellum, with lower metabolic activity in the frontal lobe.

Case 4. Parkinson's Disease with Frontotemporal Dementia:

A former English teacher in her late eighties died after two decades of Parkinson's Disease marked by slowing, gait problems and mostly inner (subjectively felt) tremor. Cognitive difficulties had progressed over the same period, but had begun a few years earlier with forgetting prior conversations. Asked about her sense of humor and any personality change, her family said that her friends had early noted a "stony face," humorlessness and lessened conversation with them, but interpreted this as her "feeling above" them. By the middle of her course, on levodopa for several years, she developed simple hallucinations of a fly on the wall without emotion. She had anxiety, but the family felt it was only when her levodopa was wearing off. She performed unusually well in the figure and clock drawing on the MoCA, and late in her course could play Scrabble. On autopsy she had at least 50% neuronal loss in her substantia nigra, consonant with her Parkinson's, no evidence of Lewy Body disease, and hippocampal and frontal lobe degenerative changes in keeping with semantic/behavioral FTD, which could explain her loss of empathy and relative insouciance that was interpreted as snobbery by her friends.

Figure: Oz characters illustrate brain differences in empathic humor

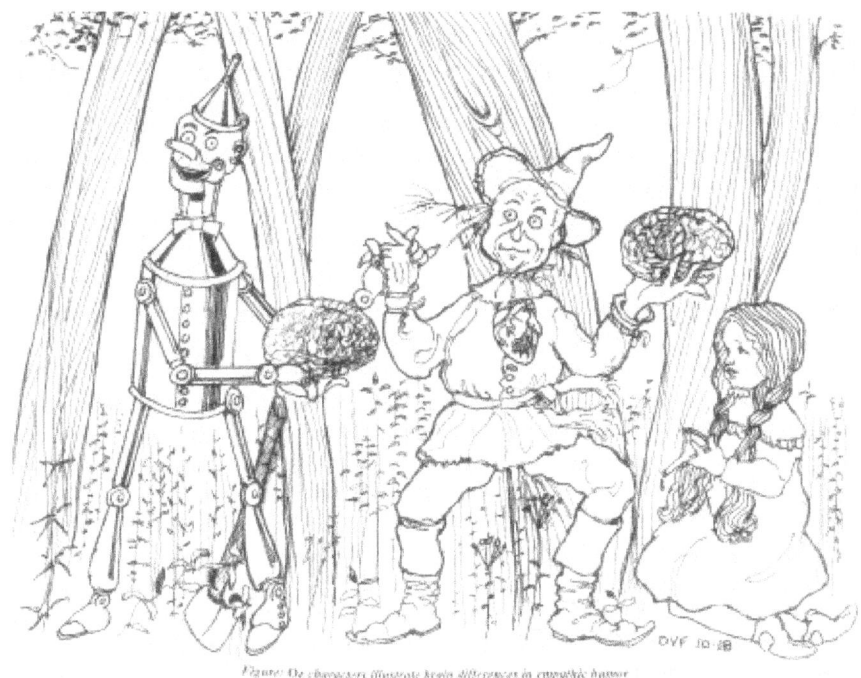

Figure: Oz characters illustrate brain differences in empathic humor

    *Setting aside pure language impairment (language variant fronto-temporal lobar degeneration, **lvFTLD**, also called primary progressive aphasia, PPA), it may be challenging diagnostically to distinguish between the behavioral variant of frontotemporal dementia, **bvFTD**, and the frontal variant of Alzheimer's disease, **fvAD**. Sawyer et al. (2017) propose as mnemonics two of Dorothy's companions along the Yellow Brick Road in L. Frank Baum's* The Wonderful Wizard of Oz *(George M. Hill Co., Chicago, 1900). Requiring different treatment and care, they are the **Scarecrow** for fvAD, brain-impaired, irritable, paranoid and tremulous; and the **Tin Man** for bvFTD, ritualistic and rigid with sometimes Parkinsonian stiffness, having more trouble with empathy, as he lacks a heart. He also, in my estimation, is lacking in a sense of humor (presciently, a bit robotic), and cannot weep lest he rust. The Tin Man may even be the prototype of the empathic limitations of half-Vulcan Mr. Spock and android Mr. Data of TV's* Star Trek.

    The difference between these types of dementia is instructive, because the Alzheimer-afflicted Scarecrow has the emotional em-

pathy to get humor, but may have trouble remembering it sufficiently if it is drawn out. The seemingly more outgoing and sometimes more inappropriately joking frontotemporal Tin Man, lacking empathy and emotional understanding, can't "get with" a joke, or laugh with comprehension and real feeling..

How to Speak With Patients and Their Families

Patients and also their family caretakers warrant caution in addressing the dementing disorders. We doctors have a motto, "First, do no harm." This means even discussing severe conditions deserves sensitivity. There are many psychosocial treatments for people with neurological disorders, whose needs often overlap with psychiatric patients, that others and I have described extensively elsewhere (Forrest, DV, 2007; Groves, M. and Forrest, DV, 2005). Suffice to say here, one may adapt how one speaks with persons whose incapacities limit communication and comprehension. Such adaptations overcome barriers to being in touch.

Adapting one's approach to various impairments:

Consciousness is usually clear in dementia, but if the person is at all obtunded, or slowed, one would speak slowly and clearly, in phrases of only a few words and a single thought at a time, continually checking for comprehension;

Attention can be variable, is also often not impaired, but if it is, distractions such as noise and clutter can be minimized to aid **registration** of cognitive input;

Retention is the main problem in dementia, requiring simplification, repetition, reinforcement by writing and diagrams, providing mnemonics, or suggesting reminder notebooks and cell phones;

Orientation to time can be helped with clocks and calendars, and scheduling visits at the same daily time;

Recognition can require self-reintroduction if one's face is not recalled, and keeping one's appearance reasonably constant between visits to aid orientation to one's person;

Construction problems may require providing external structuring, connecting cause and consequences, organizing spatial and temporal order, beginning with organizing living space, and progressing to executive function and to-do lists;

Emotion may be overly labile or flattened and impoverished; applaud measured control rather than stressing difficulties, name and feed back affects the person displays to assist verbal expression and affirm they are understood (see *Making Faces,* Forrest, 2014);

Conation problems may need support of will power but not in an overbearing or usurping manner;

Motivation when lacking can require that one facilitate positive incentives, remove impediments, and counter apathy and helplessness;

Proposition problems may require setting limits for childish opposition, encouraging nascent or half-baked positive efforts, supporting executive function, agreeing on proximate goals;

Demarcation of boundaries, if needed, may help demented persons distinguish themselves from others, especially their affects--as for example, their feelings facing family disappointment, frustration and anger.

Relation issues include interpersonal contexts and social function, and helping the caretakers to be helpful, deal with stress, fear and anger, share pleasure-- and find humor!

Plain and gentle speech: While people with dementias are owed the truth, they may be anxious about the implications. It is well to soft-pedal findings and suspected diagnoses and seek therapeutic actions to be offered. The names of some disorders may sound terrible, especially when they contain technical words. Thus, *multiple system atrophy* is a severe diagnosis one might not rush to say. Instead one might simply say "you have a Parkinson's plus disorder, which causes different problems in different folks," and focus on specific problems that can have symptomatic palliation. Sometimes explanations help, for example, "this can cause low blood pressure when you stand up, which can lead to pain across the shoulders, but it is relieved by sitting down, and we have medications that may help." Neuropsychological testing requires relaxed test conditions, and explanation of subtests: their purpose, and their relevance to the person's daily life.

Abstract or theoretical explanations are best avoided and concrete, down-to-earth language substituted, as this is easier apprehended, even by highly educated and intellectual people whose disorders and distress may render their anxious understanding more concrete. Examples: "thinned out" or "withered" for "atrophied," "aged more" for "degenerated," "trouble keeping the beat" for "dysdiadochokinesia," "losing track" for ""disoriented," "seeing things others can't see" for "hallucinations," "not caring or sharing humor so much" for "losing empathy," or "time it lasts in your body" for "halflife."

Medical jargon is best avoided whenever possible, because when people do not comprehend, they may fear the worst. Some thoughtful preparation can find substitutes, such as "forgetfulness" or "losing memories" for dementia, or "dopamine-making cells" for substantia nigra. One type of disdainful humor was to collect patients' unschooled revisions of medical language, like saying "roaches on the liver" for "cirrhosis of the liver," "fireballs in the Eucharist" for "fibroids of the uterus," and "smiling mighty Jesus" for "spinal meningitis." The joke is on us doctors when we use a medical term like cirrhosis without explaining that it means scarring of the liver. We cannot help the names of our medication, or what people think those names mean. When I was a resident psychiatrist, we had only first generation neuroleptics (antipsychotic or major tranquilizers). Taking a small survey of young adult patients' associations to the brand names of the medications they were taking, I found that Mellaril (thioridazine) sounded honey-sweet to them but, Stelazine (trifluoperazine) reminded them of stegasaurus, and Thorazine (chlorpromazine) of thunder and lightning bolts from the god Thor. A recent patient of mine with parkinsonism called levodopa "rope-a-dopa," referencing Mohmmed Ali's boxing ring technique of leaning back upon the ropes to absorb punches and tire his opponents. My patient had had an excellent result from the drug.

Once again, a person's emotional reactions is a key guide, and the leading affects can be named and reflected back to maintain rapport. Insouciance may be due to *denial,* a psychodynamic mechanism defending against realizing inner fear. On the other hand, as Edward Huey (2019) illustrated with a videotape, it may be a flattening of emotion from impairment of the frontal lobes, which appreciate emotion from the closely connected amygdala. Flattening is an emotional anesthesia, analogous to pain anesthesia, and the person with fronto-temporal dementia may truly not be feeling frightened. Frank anxiety is evidence of intactness of the frontal lobe. This good news may be shared along with cognitive and pharmacological therapies to ameliorate it. I also like to tell patients that anxiety is energy that belongs to them, which can be redirected into uses or re-channeled if overwhelming, especially into physical activities. Looking for and sharing humor about one's situation also releases tension.

Family members such as the siblings and children, may fear that they too may face the demented family member's symptoms, especially when a genetic contribution has been identified. In most cases the inherited genetic load is not the same, and genetic counseling may help. As a demented person loses awareness, the family often bears the brunt of the dementia. They may be partly consoled that, in the short time frame of the present moment, it is still possible fully to share many joys with their loved one. And living in the present moment is the prescription for happiness of the popular mindfulness movement, which aims to lessen regrets about the past or anxious worry about the future.

Appendix:

Gary Larson: empathic overextension.

John Keats (From J. Hirsh, *A Poet's Glossary*, 2014) in 1817 described the *negative capability* . With this extreme of empathy, one is "capable of being in uncertainties, Mysteries, doubts without any irritable reading after fact and reason....the displacement of the poet's protean self into another existence." Epitomizing this openness, according to Keats, was "Shakespeare [who] was the least of an egotist that it was possible to be"...and embodied "all that others were or that they could become...total immersion, for empathic release" (Keats, 1818).

Gary Larson whose cartoons are favorites of us psychiatrists, neurologists and scientists in general, deserves special attention because of his humorous and uniquely empathic approach to his subject matter with such a negative capability. Although given to a grotesquerie at times similar to fellow cartoonist Gahan Wilson, especially early in his 24-year *Far Side* series, and occasional cruelty, it is empathy that sets him apart. With absurd overextensions of a theory of mind, Larson imagines consciousnesses alien to our minds. Most often, it is the viewpoint of anthropomorphized animals who see things in species-specific ways that we do not--until he shows us. We laugh, surprised by the characterizations.

Attributing human emotions to nature or inanimate objects has been termed the **pathetic fallacy**, originally by John Ruskin in 1856, with an example from Kingsley: "They rowed her in across the rolling foam--/The cruel, crawling foam" (*Modern Painters* Vol. III, Part IV, see Cuddon, p. 493). The term is sometimes applied to the attribution of emotions to animals--but that many animals have emotions is no fallacy. Larson plays with the boundary of the pathetic fallacy and hilariously oversteps it at times.

I shall present some examples of Larson's **empathic imagination**. In a collection of his work (Larson G, 2003), the cartoons
are dated:

11-5-90 - In a restaurant frequented by giraffes, one is castigating another who has a bone stuck in his (very long) throat for being so stupid as to order fish.

11-25-90 - A spider mom with a huge pile of her eggs is phoning another to invite her over to see them, and gives her address as "Doris Griswold, 5'4", 160 lbs., brown eyes--I'm in her hair."

3-28-85 - (Even) a pregnant termite queen craves ice cream and pickles.

1-5-84 - A leopard viewing some zebras says to another that he is fed up with weeding out the sick and old and wants "something in its prime."

Against mankind's greatest fear of a post-nuclear world, depicted with mushroom clouds in each cartoon's background, three cartoons show us a non-human viewpoint:

1-4-84 - A group of insects is holding hands in a circle and dancing happily on a leaf, while nuclear clouds are visible in the background.

3-11-85 - Dogs in an underground bomb shelter are commiserating that they will have chasing squirrels no more, but "on the other hand, no more 'Fetch the stick, boy, fetch the stick.'"

9-13-85 - In the midst of a pandemonium of fires and crowds, with evacuation all around him, a dog sniffs a gutter. The caption reads, "And then Jake saw something that grabbed his attention."

Other dog cartoons explore the dog experience more lightly, yet still anthropomorphically. 2-07-85 depicts "A Dog Comedy Film Festival" with a theatre audience of rows and rows of seated dogs all wagging their tails rather than laughing or clapping.

Animals' Sense of Humor

In fact, various studies (Panksepp 2000, 2005) suggest that monkeys, dogs and even (tickled) rats laugh, using their breath and mouth in ways resembling what we do.

Larson considered animal humor in a cartoon dated 8-30-85, in which a rancher absurdly performing a card trick for a large bison is told by another rancher, "Don't play tricks on those things--they can't distinguish between 'laughing with' and 'laughing at!'"--supposing a nice distinction about bison humor, after granting them a basic sense of humor. Larson's anthropomorphizing has its limits with stolid bison!

In 2-12-85, captioned "Testing Whether Fish Have Feelings," two scientists have connected a tape deck and a microphone to a goldfish bowl, and one is insulting the goldfish as a "little bug-eyed greasy sardine! Let me tell you something about your sister!"

Species Specific Peculiarities

In 3-06-84 a snake dreams of "Free Wiener Dogs" being handed out. They are elongated, and presumably easier to swallow whole for a snake's with its own elongated body.

Larson's humor is ever a gloss upon the species-specific uniqueness of the animals' own experience, humanizing, transforming or even completely reversing what humans would expect in the same situation.

For examples, in 3-4-80 an elephant child complains to his mother about another at the table making his milk foam by blowing into it with his trunk.

And in 8-22-85, a kangaroo parent warns three young ones tucked in a bed, "Hey, you kids knock it off," and in the next panel says "That's better" when they are jumping on the bed.

Lower Phyla:

Hardly shy of moving down the ladder of the phyla, Larson takes up the insect point of view:

12-20-85 - In a forest of hairs with other fleas, one flea is carrying a sign reading "The End of the Dog Is Coming." For its readers who fear a global climate apocalypse, such 'End is Nigh' *New Yorker* cartoons are not funny, and appear rarely.

In "Last Chapter and Worse," published in 1996, the All Star Exterminators building has been struck by an Acme Chemical tank truck and the fumes have exterminated the exterminators, who are seen hanging out of the windows.

Even paramecia have consciousness, and in 3-26-85 at a cocktail party one is advising another it would be better to stay away from a third who is over by the hors d'oeuvres: "He's a nucleus-breaker" [cf. slang, "ball-buster"].

In still another, from 4-3-84, captioned "Humor at its

lowest form," one clothed amoeba is pulling on another's shirt, while punning "Shirt's on fire...NOW IT'S OUT!"

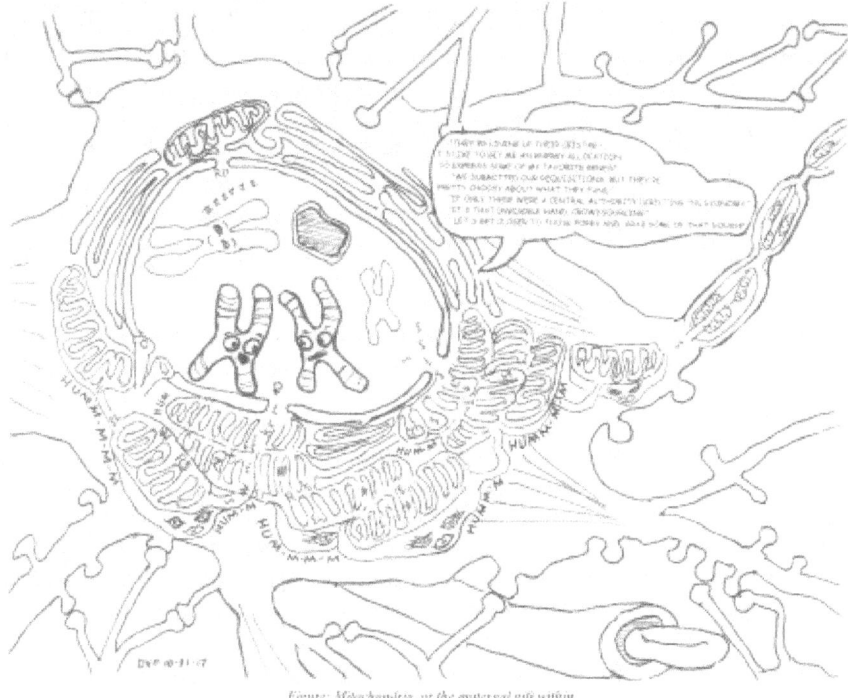

Figure: Mitochondria, or the maternal gift within

Some dementias involve poor function of the **mitochondria**, which are tiny organelles that generate energy, present in every cell except red blood corpuscles, but most important for cells that use much energy, like muscle and nervous system cells. While many mitochondrial disorders are congenital, mitochondrial dysfunction has contributed to a long list of acquired ills, including Huntington's, Alzheimer's and Parkinson's diseases, diabetes, schizophrenia, bipolar illness, anxiety disorders, and aging.

Martin Picard, Ph.D. gave a Grand Rounds at the New York State Psychiatric Institute on October 17, 2017 entitled "A Mitochondrial Link Between Brain and Body," in which he envisioned the tubule-linked mitochondrial system as nothing less than a "collectively a Lamarckian homunculus running everything."

In the illustration, the mitochondria are depicted as feminine because they are inherited exclusively through the mother's cell line.

They allocate energy, symbolized by the symbols of world currency, in ways not understood, to genes hungry to express themselves, which I have depicted as grantees seeking grants. Picard's term "homunculus" suggests they may be a coherent mental entity underlying our brain function, and his term "Lamarckian" suggests they may be able to learn and pass things on. Could they the locus of Freud's dynamic unconscious?

My including this perhaps-too-abstruse mitochondrial cartoon was prompted by Gary Larson's (4-3-84) cartoon noted just above, "Humor in its lowest form," which portrays one clothed amoeba pulling out another's shirt, punning "Shirt's on fire, now it's out." Larson's humor is having a creature at the "lowest" protozoan level of life make a pun, the so-called lowest form of humor. This requires not just getting the "fire-shirt out" pun, but the double sense of "lowest." Similarly the mitochondrial cartoon, as a burlesque at the lowest anatomical level of neuronal life, invokes some higher-level metaphorical play, and suggests that at that level, among others, mothers (via their mitochondria) again may be running things.

Even leaving the animal kingdom entirely in 7-15-85, Larson visits the question posed by its caption, "When a tree falls in the forest and no one is around," and has a conscious fallen tree musing, "Well, I'm firewood <u>now</u>! Bummer!...Say, this reminds me of a story...."

Ironically, Larson received a letter complaining about his cruelty to animals, when in fact few have done more than he to create empathy for the sentience and intelligence of animals, by his comic anthropomorphic exaggerations. He outdoes PETA! The cartoon from 12-4-81 that prompted the letter, which Larson printed next to it, depicted a herd of his impassive bison with arrows sticking out of their backs. One remarks, "Say...maybe it's not just a bad swarm of horseflies."

It is true his humor can be acerbic, if not sadistic at times. In 5-25-85 a dog with his head out of a car window happily announces to another dog he is passing that he is "going to the vet's to get tutored." One could say this cartoon has a certain pathos about the trusting innocence of pets, and that is empathic.

Similarly in 6-19-85 one cow is driving a meat truck past two other cows, and the caption reads "Eventually Murray took the job but his friends never did speak to him again."

But humans are not exempt from ironically cruel humor. In 8-2-85, A slave in a long column pullng a huge stone cube in ancient Egypt is raising his hand and complaining to the whip-wielding slave master, "Excuse me sir, but Shinkowsky keeps stepping on the back of my sandal." Even this makes us identify with a minutia of being a slave, and therefore more really. Compare Jewish humor, above.

Scientists:

Perhaps because Larson also treats scientists as the peculiar, if not alien species of human they (we) know they (we) are, scientists especially enjoy his depictions of them (us):

In a special *Science Times* feature, "The Far Side of Science," 11-24-98, one cartoon entitled "Scientist Hell" shows scientists entering a room full of people on the door of which a sign reads "Psychics, Astrologists & Mediums Eternal Discussion Group." Sorry, New Age folks, it's what we feel.

A 9-11-85 cartoon combines scientists and animal intelligence. With a doorknob on a chart and a dog pointing to it, the caption reads, "Knowing how it could change the lives of canines everywhere, the dog scientists struggled diligently to understand the Doorknob Principle."

Similarly, in 9-25-85, scientists recording porpoise speech are puzzled, and one is saying "Matthews...we're getting another one of those strange 'aw blah es span yol' sounds." (Phonetic for *habla espanol,* speak Spanish). This asks us to consider whether *maybe* other creatures don't speak *our* language.

In a classroom with formulas on the blackboard and dead scientist cats all about, the police in 9-26-85 announce, "Notice all the computations, theoretical scribblings, and lab equipment, Norm....Yes, curiosity killed these cats."

In 7-19-85, captioned "Between classes at the College of Laboratory Assistants," all the students walking about are hunchbacked (a derogatory term for those with severe kyphosis). This makes a trope of Igor, the lab assistant played by Marty Feldman in Mel Brooks' 1974 *Young Frankenstein*.

Other Sensibilities:

Larson finds a familiarity in primitive man. In 4-24-85, a clearly one-up Cro-Magnon man with a match lights a cigarette for the woman of a seated Neanderthal couple, while the Neanderthal man rubs two sticks: "Thak worked frantically to start a fire, while a Cro-Magnon man, walking erect, approached the table and simply gave Theena a light."

Clowns, distanced from us by their outlandish makeup and costumes, and (perhaps by their exaggerated facial features), often the subject of childhood phobias, are treated as another alien sensibility in need of an extension of empathy. In 2-15-84, a female clown at her door warns another clown who is holding a pie in his hand ready to throw in her face, "Hold it, not on our first date!"

And even the dead, at last, are extended a sympathetic hand. In 3-5-86, a hooded figure is turning away a salesman at the door of a cemetery wall, saying, "Sorry...we're dead."

George Booth

As exhibited in numerous *New Yorker* cartoons and the exhibit, "George Booth: A Cartoonist's Life" at The Society of Illustrators October 24, 2017 to December 30, 2017, Booth uniquely captures the dogginess and cattiness peculiar to those pets. One cartoon pictures a dog sitting inside a front door, just waiting for the return of its owner. But mostly it's the animals' apparent self-immersion in the postures and expressions of their species, oblivious to the doings of the down-and-out humans whose shabby domiciles they share, under the inevitable bare light bulb dangling on its wires from the ceiling.

"The Aristocrats"

For a hundred years, since the vaudeville era, the joke best known to comedians was like a secret handshake among them, until the ever-tasteful Gilbert Gottfried told it in 2001 at a Friar's Club roast for Hugh Hefner. Penn Jillette was at the roast, and in 2005 he made a documentary with Paul Provenza, in which 100 famous comedians vied to tell this one joke most outrageously. Dedicated to Johnny Carson, as it was said to be his favorite joke, it's such a classic that it has been called the monojoke, analogous to Joseph Campbell's (1949) monomyth about a generic legendary hero who overcomes obstacles on a cyclical journey to bring back a boon to the people, described in *The Hero With a Thousand Faces*.

The set up of this classic joke is always the same. A family comes to a theatrical agent's office to pitch their act. There is a father, a mother, a girl and a boy, and a dog.

The agent says, "Sorry, family acts are too cutesy and I've seen them all."

The father says, "Our act is unique, just give us 5 minutes and we're sure you'll agree."

"OK, 5 minutes, but no more," says the agent.

So they begin their act, which consists of outrageous pornographic and scatological behavior, including every obscene form of sex and perversion, and involving the whole family and even the dog, in such tabooed behaviors as incest, sadomasochism, coprophagia, pedophilia, bestiality, urolagnia, and so forth. Sparing the details, suffice to say deSade, Krafft-Ebing and Wilhelm Stekel might be impressed.

When they finish, the agent says, "Wow! I've never seen the likes of that. What do you call your act?"

The father stands, puffs out his chest, and proudly announces, "We call ourselves "The Aristocrats."

There are innumerable versions of the Aristocrats. Sometimes they call themselves "The Sophisticates" or "The Debonaires." It is so notorious among comedians that even mere mention of it can suffice as humor. For example, "Knock knock." "Who's there?" "The Aristocrats!" (laughter).

There's even an inverse Aristocrats. In the documentary, Wendy Liebman delivers her inverse version in a sweet, soft voice: The family are the Cavanaughs, Anne and William. They have two children, Betsy and Timmy. They are finishing dinner, and as the maid clears the plates, Anne suggests the family go into the drawing room, where Anne braids little Betsy's beautiful blonde hair, William plays chess with Timmy, and the maid comes in with a plate of strawberries and cream. They all have a nice dessert.

"What do you call your act?" the agent asks.

"The C-----------g M-----------s!"

The cognitive function necessary to understand this seeming race to the bottom by all the professional comedians in The Aristocrats includes acknowledging the over-the-top outrageous exaggerations in the various versions which are not, in themselves, very funny. "The Aristocrats" is not a dirty joke; it is a basic script for a virtuoso improvisation. Inasmuch as it is about irony, it belongs under that rubric above. A sophistication is required to permit the cognitive distance neither to be shocked nor fascinated by the obscenities, and rather to see the film as a mock battle in the linguistic realm, in which timing and other delivery skills can be flaunted.

"The Aristocrats" comedians were setting aside their reactions to the atrocity to appreciate the joke's irony, as well as the performative virtuosity each was vying to top. Simply being shocked by the obscenities or taboo acts or, worse, being amused or fascinated by them per se, would be to miss the point. The listener must be able to avoid and be unaffected by the emotion (isolate the affect), which is an inhibitory capacity, a mental strength. The joke contrasts obscenity with a play on the idea of being classy. Rather than being about obscenity, it is on a mental level apart from titillation.

A patient with diminished frontal lobe function might lose this inhibitory process One of my patients and his very aged father play-mimicked the screamed orders of the Nazis they both had survived. I was apprehensive (needlessly, it turned out) that if his father ever suffered this kind of cognitive decline (which to his death he did not), his comprehension of the comedic framework might be lost and the horrific tones taken as authentic rather than play.

Glee about just pronouncing taboo words, independent of context, is associated with emotional immaturity and the stage of pre-adolescence that cherishes fart jokes. To make a sweeping generalization, people of higher intelligence and self-control tend to be better able to distance themselves from emotional reactivity and to view the content of humor dispassionately, even when it is shockingly off-color. I realize my contention is being tested on the campuses with their trigger words and safe spaces, but losing track of the context (historical, analytical or whatever humorous intent) upon feeling horror about any particular word is a mental limitation, even if it is a posture taught and learned.

To return to my previous anecdote about the Mensa meeting I observed, there was music, but no one danced; a pool, but no one swam--instead having races with boats made of popsicle sticks and rubber bands. They sure were playing the part of nerds. But when they assembled, they had an open joke session, and I have seldom heard such a run of offensive, but really funny dirty jokes, delivered without much audible emotional reaction. Their seemingly purely intellectual appreciation was neither a childish relishing of scatology or a smirking at the dirty jokes.

Much as "The Aristocrats" contemplates the violative as a construct, these highly intelligent Mensa members were comparing their jokes dispassionately. I had spent the afternoon with them and had no reason to doubt their decency, fairness, sensitivity and other virtues one would like to think come with intelligence (but not always; it's a cliché that the cinema is rife with villains of high intelligence and taste). "The Aristocrats" is not about sex or sexuality, and the comedians in Jillette's documentary were not sex offenders. Granted that some smart people who lack empathy could wallow in the scatology, or have a mentality unfiltered by the distance of emotional control, being limited to a brutish level of obscenity may reflect character limitations or neuropsychiatric pathology.

Once again, getting low-level humor does not consign one to being rated at a low level of capacity--unless the low level is the *only* level of humor to which one responds.

Relationships and Unsteadiness on One's Feet

Figure: The Fahn pull test

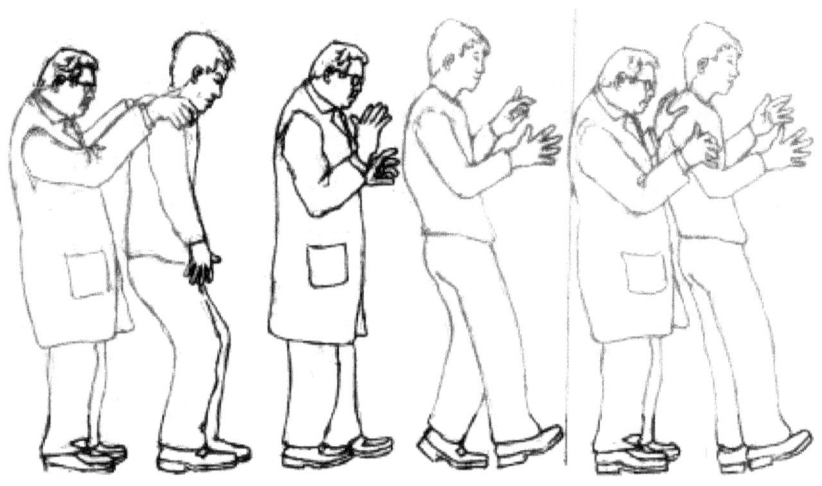

Figure: The Fahn pull test

Unsteadiness of the feet (abasia) can lead to emotional insecurity in our patients. An academic psychology experiment (Forest AL, 2015) found that 47 neurologically intact volunteers (18 male, 29 female, mean age 21) who stood on one foot compared to two feet, or sat on unstable chairs, also rated their romantic relationships as less secure ("how satisfied they felt with their partner and whether they thought the relationship would last"). Forest was attempting to model (in a minor way) the effects of an earthquake, such as in Sichuan in 2008, including a higher rate of divorce that followed that natural catastrophe.   A similar literal-into-abstract translation occurs in conditions with unsteadiness on the feet, such as Parkinsonism or (more common) vestibular disorders. People who are unsteady on their feet feel fearful and are vulnerable to cruel ridicule, mockery and the implication of inebriation.

Cases: A businesswoman in her late 70's with imbalance from vestibular impairment from an antibiotic, and a retired investor in his 80's who developed imbalance from neuropathic problems and Parkinson's disease, both developed serious doubts about their spouses that were relieved, in the first case with instruction how to walk and turn while keeping the head steady and fixing the gaze like a pirouetting ballerina; and in the second case, by supportive psychotherapy and levodopa.

The Pull Test *(Fahn, et al., 1987, Munhoz, et a. 2014) is a reassuring and trust-building maneuver to evaluate postural stability. The procedure is explained and the test is the person's response to a sudden pull back on shoulders from standing with eyes open and feet slightly apart. These are the ratings from the Unified Parkinson's Disease Rating Scale:*

0 = Normal: requires 0-2 steps backward to regain balance
1 = Retropulsion,that is, backwards steppage, but recovers unaided after more than 2 backward steps
2 = Absence of postural response; would fall (like a log) if not caught by examiner
3 = Very unstable, tends to lose balance spontaneously
4 = Unable to stand without assistance.

The Pull Test is practical because it evaluates recovery from induced backward imbalance, a real-life risk. Moreover, it quantifies the unsteadiness which, like tremor, often triggers cruel ridicule.

List of logical mechanisms (Attardo, 2001, p.27)

This fascinating list invites perusing of its source for elaboration:

Role reversals, vacuous reversal, garden path, almost situations, inferring consequences, coincidence, proportion, exaggeration, meta-humor, role exchanges, juxtaposition, figure-ground reversal, analogy, reasoning from false premise, parallelism, ignoring the obvious, field restriction, vicious circle, potency mappings, chiasmus, faulty reasoning, self-undermining, missing link, implicit parallelism, false analogy, cratylism [a naturalistic theory of language that names have a direct link with their meaning--as for example in onomatopoeia-- rather than being arbitrary signs], referential ambiguity.

The 5 most common [logical] oppositions (Attardo, 2001, p. 20) are: Good/bad, life/death, obscene/non-obscene, money/no money/ high/low stature. These figure in a lot of jokes.

List of Women Comedians (see **Rating** of -0 to -1, Targets of Humor and Butts of Jokes, above). The term comedians is preferred to comediennes. There have been very funny women on stage for more than a century:
Fanny Brice (1891-1951)
Moms Mabley (1894-1975), the first female stand-up comedian
Gracie Allen (1895-1964)
Imogene Coca (1908-2001)
Lucille Ball (1911-89)
Minnie Pearl (1912-96)
Phyllis Diller (1917-2012)
Bea Arthur (1922-2009)
Audrey Meadows (1922-96)
Betty White (1922-)
Totie Fields (1930-1978)
Elaine May (1932-)
Carol Burnett (1933-)
Joan Rivers (1933-2014)
Carol Burnett (1933-)
Joanne Worley (1937-)
Lily Tomlin 1939-)

Madeline Kahn (1942-99)
Penny Marshall (1943-2018)
Goldie Hawn (1945-
Bette Midler (1945-)
Roseanne Barr (1951-)
Whoopie Goldberg (1955-)
Ellen DeGeneres (1958-)
Kathy Griffin (1960-)
Julia Louis-Dreyfus (1961-)
Rosie O'Donnell (1962-)
Wanda Sykes (1964-)
Leslie Jones (1967-)
Margaret Cho (1968-)
Jane Krakowski (1968-)
Melissa McCarthy (1970-)
Tina Fey (1970-)
Sarah Silverman (1970-)
Amy Poehler (1971-)
Kristin Wiig (1973-)
Mayim Bialik (1975-)
Gilda Radner (1946-89)
Amy Schumer (1981-)
Ms. Pat (1972-)

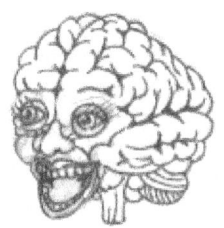

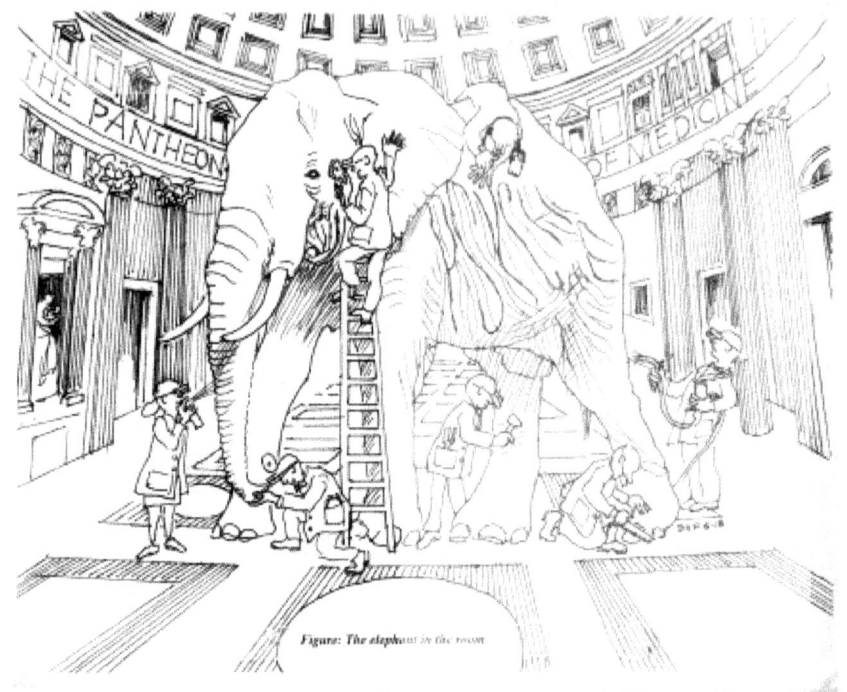

Figure 15: The elephant in the room

The whole is more. A sense of humor is a part of us. It is of great social, expressive and restorative value, but it is just a part, and needs to be considered in its context of ourselves and our social selves, as it so often is a basis for our relationships. This final illustration, which my neurologist colleagues liked and pinned to the wall of the doctors' station of our Movement Disorders Clinic, depicts clinical medicine addressing the perpetual problem of grasping the elephant in the room. In the original parable, blind men investigate an elephant by touch, and one, feeling the trunk, deems it a snake; one who feels an elephant leg, thinks it's a tree trunk, and so forth. In the cartoon, the blind men are medical specialists who risk seeing only a portion of the whole patient while giving care. Meanwhile, written on the elephant's side in letters that are not seen at first, like theatre cartoonist Al Hirschfeld's embedded name of his daughter Nina, is the patient's psyche, which contributes to every step the patient takes from initial presentation to treatment.

References:

Abrams R (2019): Serious business at the Friars Club, *The New York Times* April 14, 2019.

Acharya S and Shukla S (2012): Mirror neurons: enigma of the metaphysical modular brain, *Journal of Natural Science, Biology and Medicine,* v.3(2):118-124, Jul-Dec 2012.

Ajaye F (2002): *Comic Insights: The Art of Stand-up Comedy*, Beverly Hills, Los Angeles, Silman-James Press.

Apperly IA, Samson D, Chiavarino C and Humphreys GW (2004): Frontal and temporo-parietal lobe contributions to theory of mind: neuropsychological evidence from a false-belief task with reduced language and executive demands, *J. Cogn. Neurosci.* 16:1773-1783. doi:10.1162/0898929042947928.

Amira D (2018): Jerry Seinfeld says jokes are not real life, *The New York Times,* August 15, 2018.

Associated Press (2019): April fools: Robots still don't get the joke, April 2019.

Attardo S (2001): *Humorous Texts: A Semantic and Pragmatic Analysis*, Berlin and New York, Mouton de Gruyter.

Attardo S and Raskin V (1991): Script theory revisited: joke similarity and like representation model, *Humor* 4:293-347. doi:10.1515/humr.1991.4.3-4.293.

Baker G (2019): The strangely dovish Donald Trump, *The Wall Street Journal Review,* Saturday/Sunday July 6-7, 2019, p. C2.

Barry D (2019): *Lessons From Lucy: The Simple Joys of an Old Happy Dog,* New York, Simon and Schuster.

Bardon M (1931): *'Don Quichotte' en France au XVIIe et au XVIIIe siécle, 1605-1815,* 2 vols. (Paris, 1931), I, iii.

Bergson H (1900, 1924): *Le Rire: Essai sur la Signication du Comique,* published as 3 essays in *Revue de Paris* in 1900 and in 1924 as a book of the same title, which is translated as *Laughter: On he Meaning of the Comic,* Paris, Alcan, 1924.

Berman E (2014): Song of the Day--"Alice's Restaurant Massacre" by Arlo Guthrie Booth Reviews, Chicagonow.com. Retrieved 2 Jun 2014 (Wikipedia).

Bettelheim B (1976): *The Uses of Enchantment: The Meaning and Importance of Fairy Tales,* London and New York, Thames & Hudson.

Bijanki KR, Manns JR, Inman CS, Choi KS, Harati S, Pedersen NP, Drane DL, Waters AC, Fasano RE, Mayberg HS, Willie JT (2019): Cingulum stimulation enhances positive affect and anxiolysis to facilitate awake craniotomy, *J. Clin Invest* 2019 Mar 1; 129(3):1152-1166. doi:10.1172/JCI120110 Epub 2019 Feb 11. See also Mills KA (2019): Probing the happy place, J Clin Invest 2019 Mar 1; 129(3):1952-1954.

Binsted K and Ritchie G (1994): An implemented model of punning in riddles, *Proceedings of the Twelfth National Conference on Artificial Intelligence (AAA 1-94),* Seattle, USA.

Birnbach L (1980): *The Official Preppy Handbook,* New York, Workman Publishing Company.

Björnsdotter M, Wang M, Pelphrey K, Kaiser MD (2016): Evaluation of quantified social perception circuit activity as a neurobiological marker of autism spectrum disorder, *JAMA Psychiatry.* 2016;73(6):614-621, June 2016.

Bloom P (2016): *Against Empathy: The Case for Rational Compassion,* New York, Ecco/HarperCollins, described in Shai Held, The most overrated virtue, *The Wall Street Journal,* January 3, 2017, A25.

Bond, Simon (1988): *101 Uses for a Dead Cat,* New York, Clarkson Potter, 2 Nov 1988.

Bowser AD (2019): 'Pathway to dementia:' Alzheimer's - like disorder hits in LATE life, *Clinical Pathology News,* p. 1, 6-7, June 2019.

Brockman DD Sr. (2017): *A Psychoanalytic Exploration of Dante's* The Divine Comedy, London and New York, Routledge/Taylor & Francis Group.

Brooks D (2018): In search of the perfect joke, *The New York Times Magazine,* 9/2/18, pp. 42-45, 50.

Belluck P (2018): Will we ever cure Alzheimer's? *The New York Times/Science Times,* November 20, 2018, p. D2.

Campbell J (1949): *The Hero With a Thousand Faces*, New York, Pantheon.

Cao H, Bertolino A, Walter H, et al. (2016): Altered functional subnetwork during emotional face processing: a potential intermediate phenotype for schizophrenia, *JAMA Psychiatry* 2016;73(6):598-605, June 2016.

Castellanos S (2019): A tech nerd walks into a bar...: Campus requires improv class for computer scientists, *The Wall Street Journal* May 5, 2019, pp. 1,19.

Cazala F, Vienney N, and Stoleru S (2015): The cortical sensory representation of genitalia in women and men: a systematic review, *Socioaffect Neurosci Psychol.* 2015; 5:10.340/snp.v5.26428. Published online 2015 Mar10 doi: 10.3402/snp.v5.26428.

Cepelewicz J (2019): How the brain creates a timeline of the past: The brain can't directly encode the passage of time, but recent work hints at workaround for putting timestamps on memories of events, *Quanta Magazine.* February 12, 2019.

Chan Y-C, Lavallee JP (2015): Temporo-parietal and fronto-parietal lobe contributions to theory of mind and executive control: an fMRI study of verbal jokes, *Frontiers in Psychology* 2015;6:1285, published online 2915 Sep 2.doi: 10:3389/fpsyq.2015.01285.

Chute H (2017): *Why Comics? From Underground to Everywhere,* New York, HarperCollins. The Modern Language Association published a cluster of critical articles about Chute's book, *PMLA* 134.3, pp. 569-637, Theories and Methodologies.

Clark, Camilla et al. (2015): Altered sense of humor in dementia, *Journal of Alzheimer's Disease* 49(1)111-119, 2015.

Corsellis JA, Bruton CJ, Freeman-Browne D (1973): The aftermath of boxing, *Psychological Medicine* 3:270-303.

Corhallis MC (2011): *The Recursive Mind: The Origins of Language, Thought and Civilization,* Princeton, N.J., Princeton University Press.

Cooper H, Baker P, Schmitt E, and Ferman M (2018): 2 years in, still struggling to understand 'my military,' *The New*

York Times, International, Saturday November 17, 2018, p. A12.

Cousins N (1979): *Anatomy of an Illness as Perceived by a Patient: Reflections on Healing and Regeneration,* introduction by Rene Dubos, New York, Norton.

Cuddon JA (1979): *A Dictionary of Literary Terms,* New York, Penguin 1976, 1977, 1979.

Cummings EE (1991): *Complete Poems 1904-1962,* edited by George Firmage, New York, Liveright.

Cunningham V (2019): What are you laughing at? Tracy Morgan turns the drama of his life into comedy again, *The New Yorker,* May 13, 2019, p. 38.

Dante A (1308): *The Divine Comedy, Inferno, Purgatory, Paradise.* Trans. C.S. Singleton (1973), Bollingen Series LXXX, Princeton, N.J., Princeton University Press.

Darling J (2002): Humor: a coping strategy for pediatric patients, *Pediatric Nursing* 28(2)123-131, Jan 2002.

Dauber J (2017): *Jewish Comedy: A Serious History,* , New York, Norton.

Dawkins R (1976): *The Selfish Gene,* Oxford, England, UK, Oxford University Press.

Devetak R (1995/1996): Postmodernism, pp. 170-209 in Burchill S and Linklater A, *Theories of International Relations,* New York, St. Martins, p.184.

Dickson P (1984,1986): *Too Much Saxon Violence,* New York, Dell Publishing Co.

Diffee M (2011): *The Best of the Rejection Collection: 293 Cartoons That Were Too Dumb, Too Dark, or Too Naughty for The New Yorker,* with a foreword by Robert Mankoff, the magazine's cartoon editor. New York, Workman Publishing.

Dryden, John (2013): *The Delphi Complete Works of John Dryden (Illustrated),* Hastings, U.K. Delphi Classics.

Dubois B, Slachevsky A, Litvan I and Pillon B (2000): The FAB: A frontal assessment battery at bedside, *Neurology* 55:1621-1626, December (1 of 2), 2000.

Dundes, Alan (1987): "That's Not Funny--That's Sick/ Folklorist Alan Dundes looks at the serious side of sick jokes," *St.*

Petersburg Times, 2 December 1987.

Eagleton T (2019a): The politics of humor: Whose laughter? Which comedy?, *Commonwealth,* May 6, published May 17, 2019, v.146n.9. See also Swaim B, review of *Humour,* (2019) by Terry Eagleton, New Haven, Yale, in *The Wall Street Journal,* June 7, 2019, p. A13.

Eagleton T (2019b): *Humour,* New Haven and London, Yale University Press.

Epstein J (2019): The long, sad descent of "staircase wit," *The Wall Street Journal,* Opinion Page, January 18, 2019.

Fahn, S., Elton, R.L., & UPDRS program members (1987). Unified Parkinson's Disease Rating Scale. In Fahn S, Marsden CD, Goldstein M, Caine DB, editors, *Recent Developments in Parkinson's Disease* vol. 2, Florham Park, N.J., Macmillan Healthcare Information, pp. 153-163, 293-304.

Federle T (2013): *Tequila Mockingbird: Cocktails With a Literary Twist,* Philadelphia, Running Press.

Federle T (2015): *Gone With the Gin: Cocktails With a Hollywood Twist, Tequila Mockingbird: Cocktails With a Literary Twist,* Philadelphia, Running Press.

Federle T (2018): *Are You There God? It's Me, Margarita: More Cocktails With a Literary Twist,* Philadelphia, Running Press.

Filippelli M, Pellegrio R, Iandelli I, Misuri G Rodarte JR, Duranti R, Brusasco V, and Scano G (1985): Respiratory dynamics during laughter, *J. Appl. Physiol.* (1985)2001 Apr, 90(4):1441-6.

Forest AL, Kille DR, Wood JV, Stehouwer LR (2015): Turbulent times, rocky relationships: Relational consequences of experiencing physical instability, *Psychological Science,* published online June 25, 2015.

Forrest DV (1960): The Motions of Meaning in the Poetry of E. E. Cummings, unpublished senior thesis in the Department of English, at Firestone Library, Princeton, N.J., Princeton University.

Forrest DV (1965): Poiesis and the Language of Schizophrenia, *Psychiatry* 28:1-18.

Forrest DV (1971): Vietnamese Maturation: The Lost Land of Bliss, *Psychiatry* 34:111-139.

Forrest DV (1974): *Selected American Expressions (for the Foreign-Born Psychiatrist and Other Professionals, With Street Slang Supplement)*, Revised 1976, 1982. New York, Educational Research.

Forrest DV (1976): Nonsense and sense in schizophrenic language, *Schizophrenia Bulletin* 9(2):286-301.

Forrest DV (1987): Dreams of the Rarebit Fiend: Neuromedical synthesis of unconscious meaning, *Journal of the American Academy of Psychoanalysis* 15:3:331-363.

Forrest DV (2002): Afterword to *Krazy*: George Herriman's *Krazy Kat* Cartoon and Its Appeal to E.E. Cummings, *Journal of the American Academy of Psychoanalysis* 30:2:249-258, Summer 2002.

Forrest DV (2007): Psychotherapy for patients with neuropsychiatric disorders, chapter in *The American Psychiatric Publishing Textbook of Neuropsychiatry and Clinical Neurosciences*, Fifth Edition, Edited by Yudofsky SC and Hales RE, Washington, D.C., American Psychiatric Publishing.

Forrest DV (2012): *SLOTS: Praying to the God of Chance*, Harrison, N.Y. and Encino, CA, Delphinium /OpenRoadMedia /HarperCollins.

Forrest, DV (2014). *Making Faces: Facial Emotion Workout Video.* http://vimeo.com/makingfaces/neurologic. For designated patient and medical audiences. Password: faces.

Forrest DV (2017): *Beyond Eden: The Other Lives of Fine Arts Models and The Meaning of Medical Disrobing*, Denver, CO, Outskirts Press.

Freud S (1905) [trans. 1960 by J. Strachey]: *Der Witz und Seine Beziehung zum Unbewussten*, published in Austria and Germany by F. Deuticke.

Freud S (1928): Humor, *Imago 14*, trans. Joan Rivere (1928) *Int J Psycho-Anal., Collected Papers, Vol 5*, pp. 215-221, ed. James Strachey, New York, Basic Books, 1959.

Fussell P (1983): *Class: A Guide Through the American Sta-*

tus System, New York, Simon & Schuster. See also ST Loh, Class dismissed: American status anxiety is infecting affluent hipdom, *The Atlantic* March 2009.

Geary J (2018): *Wit's End: What Wit Is, How It Works and Why We Need It*, New York, Norton. Reviewed by Henry Hitchings, *Wall Street Journal* Nov 10-11., 2018.

Gervais R (2019): I've got enough F----ing Golden Globes money! *The Hollywood Reporter*, January 3, 2020, pp. 60-64.

Gorey E (1961): *The Hapless Child*, New York, Obolensky.

Gorey E (1963): *The Gashlycrumb Tinies*, New York, Simon & Schuster.

Gopnik A (2016): Feel me: What the new science of touch says about ourselves, *The New Yorker,* May 16, 2016, pp. 56-66.

Groves M and Forrest DV, (2005): Psychiatric aspects of Parkinson's disease as a model for chronic neurodegenerative disease, in Karen Anderson, William Weiner and Anthony Wang, *Behavioral Neurology of Movement Disorders*, Philadelphia, Lippincott Williams & Wilkins, 2005.

Harris EA (2019): Amy Schumer, Ali Wong and the rise of pregnant standup, *The New York Times*, April 20, 2019, pp. C1,C4.

Heller N (2018): San Jose Postcard: Real Talk, *The New Yorker*, September 10, 2018, p.39.

Hillman J and Boer C (1985): *Freud's Own Cookbook*, Illustrated by Jeff Fisher, New York, Harper Colophon Books, Harper & Row.

Hirsh, Edward (2014): *A Poet's Glossary*, New York, Houghton Mifflin.

Hitchens C (2011) Christopher Hitchens on the true spirit of Christmas, *Wall Street Journal* December 24, 2011, Review Section (www.wsj.com/articles/SBI00014205297020--4791104577110880255067656).

Hoche F, Guell X, Vangel MG. Sherman JC and Schmahmann JD (2018): The cerebellar cognitive affective /Schmahmann syndrome scale, *Brain* 1411248-270 (Jan 1).

Hoberman J and Shandler J (2003): *Entertaining America: Jews, Movies and Broadcasting,* New York, The Jewish Museum, and Princeton, N.J., Princeton University Press.

Homskaya, Evgenia D (2001): *Alexander Romanovitch Luria: A Scientific Biography*, New York, Springer.

Hofstadter, Douglas R (1979): *Goedel, Escher, Bach: An Eternal Golden Braid,* New York, Basic Books.

Howard MW, Eichenbaum H (2013): The hippocampus, time and memory across scales, *J Experimental Psychology: General* 142:4:1211.

Huey ED (2019): Paradigm shifts in neurodegenerative disorders, Columbia Psychiatric Grand Rounds June 5, 2019.

Iannone C (2018): Seinfeld: The politically incorrect comedy, *Modern Age: A Conservative Review*, Vol 60 No 2, Spring 2018.

Ingvar DH, Franzen G (1974): Abnormalities of cerebral blood flow distribution in patient with chronic schizophrenia, *Acta Psychiatrica Scandinavica* 50(4)425-462.

Jaffe J, Beebe B, Feldstein S, Crown CL and Jasnow MD (2002): *Rhythms of Dialogue in Infancy*, Boston, Blackwell,

James H (1983): *The Aspern Papers and Other Stories*, Edited with an introduction and notes by Adrian Poole, New York, Oxford University Press, introduction p. xv.

Kaplan M (2018): Biopic of drunk, damaged and darkly hilarious artist, *The New York Post,* July 12, 2018, pp. 20-21.

Kandel ER (2018): *The Disordered Mind: What Unusual Brains Tell Us About Ourselves,* New York, Farrar, Straus and Giroux.

Kaldun A, et al. (2016): Observing the ultrafast buildup of a Fano resonance in the time domain, *Science* 354:738-747.

Kalin NH (2019): Prefrontal cortical and limbic circuit alterations in psychopathology, *American Journal of Psychiatry* 176:12: 97-973.

Katz M (1999, 2010) *Jewish as a Second Language: How to Worry, How to Interrupt, How to Say the Opposite of What You Mean.* Illustrated by Jeff Moores, New York, Workman Publishing.

Keller H (1905): *The Story of My Life.* Mineola, N.Y., Dover

Thrift Edition, 1996.

Kendler K (2018): The development of Kraepelin's mature diagnostic concepts of paranoia (Die Verrücktheit) and paranoid dementia praecox (dementia paranoides): A close reading of his textbooks from 1887 to 1899, *JAMA Psychiatry* 75(12):1280-1288.

Kipps CM, Nestor PJ, Acosta-Cabronero J, Arnold R, Hodges JR (2009): Understanding social dysfunction in the behavioral variant of frontotemporal dementia: the role of emotional sarcasm processing, *Brain,* 132;3:592-603, 06 Jan 09. 1 Mar 09.

Komisaruk BR, Wise N, Frangos E, Liu WC, Allen K, Brody S (2011): Women's clitoris, vagina and cervix mapped on the sensory cortex: fMRI evidence, *Journal of Sexual Medicine* Oct 8(10):2822-30.

Kraepelin E (1896): *Psychiatrie: Ein Lehrbuch fuer Studierende und Aerzte,* Leipzig, Fuenfte, Vollstaendig umgearbeitete Auflage.

Larson G (2003): *The Complete Far Side, Vol. One, 1980-1986* and *Volume Two, 1987-1994,* Marietta/Atlanta, GA 30141, Lionheart Books, Ltd.

Levin F (2009): *Emotion and the Psychodynamics of the Cerebellum; A Neuro-Analytic Analysis and Synthesis,* ,London, Karnac Books,

Lieberman JA, Small SA, and Girgis RR (2019): Early detection and preventive intervention in schizophrenia: From fantasy to reality, *Am J Psychiatry* 176:794-810.

Lieberman R (2018): Glamour wounds, *The Rhonda Lieberman Reader*, edited and published by Sarah Lehrer-Grainer, L.A. Pep Talk 7.

Lifton RJ (1982): Beyond psychic numbing: a call for awareness, *American Journal of Orthopsychiatry* 52(4).

Lupton E and Lipps A (1918): *The Senses: Design Beyond Vision,* New York, Cooper Hewitt, Smithsonian Design Museum and Princeton, N.J., Princeton University Architectural Press.

Mainwaring M (2019): Deconstructing the tutu: is ballet

camp? *The New York Times,* May 29, 2019, p. C7.

Malcolm J (1981): *The Impossible Profession,* New York, Knopf.

Marshall A (2015): A robot walks into a bar, but can it do comedy? *The New York Times,* August 8, 2015.

Martin W (2015): *The Primates of Park Avenue: A Memoir: Inside the Secret Sisterhood of Manhattan Moms,* New York, Simon & Schuster.

Mayeux R, Ottman R, Maestre G et al. (1995): Synergistic effects of traumatic head injury and apoprotein-epsilon 4 on patients with Alzheimer's disease, *Neurology* 45:555-557.

McGhee P (1979): *Humor: Its Origin and Development,* San Francisco, W.H. Freeman.

Mendelsohn D (2016): How Greek drama saved the city, *The New York Review* June 23, 2016, pp. 59-61.

Michl P, Meindl T, Meister F, Born C, Engel RR, Reiser M and Hennig-Fast K (2014): Neurobiological underpinnings of shame and guilt: a pilot fMRI study, Social Cognitive and Affective Neuroscience, Vol 9, Issue 2,1, February 2014, pp. 150-157.

Mitchell H (2019): What can science tell us about dad jokes? *The Wall Street Journal,* 28 Feb 19, p. A11.

Mochizuki H (2014): Brain processing of itching and scratching, Ch. 23 in *Itch: Mechanisms and Treatment,* Carstens E and Akiyama T, eds., Philadelphia, CRC Press/Taylor and Francis.

Munhoz RP, Li J-Y, Kurtinecz M, Piboolnurak P, Constantino A, Fahn S, Lang AE (2004) Evaluation of the pull test technique in assessing postural instability in Parkinson's Disease, *Neurology* 62(1):125-127, Jan 13, 2004.

Nagel T (2018): As if!, *The New York Review of Books,* pp. 36-40, April 5, 2018.

Nash O (1995): *Selected Poetry of Ogden Nash: 650 Rhymes, Verses, Lyrics and Poems,* Introduction by Archibald MacLeish, New York, Black Dog and Leventhal.

Nelson PT, Dickson RW, Trojanowski JQ, Jack CR, Boyle PA, Arfanakis K (2019): *Brain* 142(6) 1503-1527, Jun 1; April

30. doi:10.1093/brain/awz099.

Newton BW et al. (2008): Is there hardening of the heart during medical school? *Academic Medicine* 83(3)244-249, March 2008.

Novak W and Waldoks M (1981): *The Big Book of Jewish Humor*, New York, HarperCollins.

Oates JC (2018): Proust questionnaire, *Vanity Fair Holiday 2018-2019 Issue*, p. 134.

Panksepp J (2000): The riddle of laughter: neural and psychoevolutionary underpinnings of joy, *Current Directions in Psychological Science* 9(6).doi:10.1111/1467-8721.00090.

Panksepp J (2005): No joke: animals laugh too, *Science* March 21, 2005, www.livescience.com/6946-joke-animals-laugh-html.

Parker G (2016): Psychiatrists as cartoon characters: how the *New Yorker* has traced psychiatry over the decades, *American Journal of Psychiatry* 173:9:875, September 2016.

Penfield W and Boldrey E (1937): Somatic motor and sensory representation in the cerebral cortex of man as studied by electrical stimulation, *Brain* 60:389-443 doi:10.1093/brain/60.4.389.

Penfield W and Rasmussen T (1950):*The Cerebral Cortex of Man*, New York, Macmillan.

Perelman SJ (1947): *The Best of S.J. Perelman*, New York, Random House, The Modern Library.

Piaget J (1962): *Play, dreams and imitation in childhood*, New York, Norton.

Pierce M (2016): A joke in your brain from the start to the punchline, *Brain Candy*, 16 October 2015, online at https://braindecoder.com/post/neuroscience-of-humor-1407626439, 4/18/2016.

Pinker S (2011): *The Better Angels of Our Nature: Why Violence Has Declined*, New York, Viking.

Powell T (2019): *Dementia Re-imagined*, New York, Avery-Penguin Random House.

Provine RP (2000): *Laughter: A Scientific Investigation*,

New York, Penguin.

Rafil MS and Santoro SL (2018): Prevalence and severity of Alzheimer's disease in individuals with Down syndrome, *JAMA Neurol* published online Nov 19, 2018, doi:10.1001/JAMA Neurol 2018.3443.

Radtke OL (2007): *Chinglish: Found in Translation*, Layton, Utah, Gibbs Smith, 2007.

Rowsome F, Jr. (1965): *The Verse by the Side of the Road: The Story of the Burma-Shave Signs and Jingles*, with drawings by Carl Rose, Brattleboro, Stephen Greene Books.

Salwen, B (1946): For nofur trunnions, *Time* 15 April 1946.

Sandomir R (2018): Will Jordan, 91, Comedian Who Mimicked the Famous, *The New York Times*, obituaries, September 11, 2018.

Sarnoff CA (1976): *Latency*, New York, Jason Aronson.

Sawyer RP, Rodrigues-Porcel F, Hagen M, Shatz R, Espay AJ (2017): Diagnosing the frontal variant of Alzheimer's disease: a clinician's yellow brick road, *J. Clin Mov Dis* 2017 Mar 2; 4:2.

Schine C (2017): So funny you could plotz, review of Jeremy Dauber, Jewish Comedy: A Serious History, *The New York Review of Books*, March 8, 2018,

Schwab N and Moore M (2019): Trump and Pelosi go nuts on each other, *The New York Post*, May 24, 2019, pp. 8-9.

Shanor K and Kanwal J (2911): *Bats Sing, Mice Giggle*, London, Icon Books.

Shankar K, Singh I, Howard MH (2016): Neural mechanism to simulate a scale-invariant future timeline, *Neural Computation* 28:2594-2627.

Shaw H (1972): *Dictionary of Literary Terms*, New York, McGraw-Hill.

Sherrington (1942): *Man on His Nature*, Cambridge, U.K., Cambridge University Press, p. 178.

Small SA, Schobel SA, Buxton RB, et al. (2011): A pathophysiologicl framework of hippocampal dysfunction in ageing and disease, *Nat Rev Neurosci* 12:585-601.

Sontag S (1964): Notes on camp, *Partisan Review* 31(4) 515-530, Fall 1964. Reprinted as *Notes on Camp* (2018), New York, Penguin Random House.

Strauss GP, Nunez A, Ahmed AO, Barchard KA, Granholm E, Kirkpatrick B, Gold JM, and Allen DN (2018): The latent structure of negative symptoms in schizophrenia, *JAMA Psychiatry* 75(12):1271-1279.

Stetson L (1976): *The Ballet Company Game*, New York, Stetson Enterprises, New York. The classic board game from the Balanchine era, available from Lynne Stetson Forrest, 155 West 68th Street, Suite 1219, New York, New York 10023, or contact davidvforrest@gmail.com.

Stone MH (2009): *The Anatomy of Evil*, Amherst, New York, Prometheus.

Strogatz SH (2004): *Sync: How Order Emerges From Chaos in the Universe, Nature and Daily Life*, New York, Hachette.

Swarner K (1996): *Yiddish Wisdom: Yiddishe Chochma,* San Franciso, Chronicle Books.

Verplaste J (2009): *Localizing Moral Sense: Neuroscience and the Sense of Morality 1800-1930*, Springer, New York.

Weaver S (2019): Spirit of 'camp' is in fashion at Met,' *am New York*, May 7, 2019, p. 9.

Wells G and Horwitz J (2019): Content factories swamp Instagram, diluting its appeal, *The Wall Street Journal* September 27, 2019, pp. A1,A9.

Weems S (2018): On sick humor and the art of laughing at tragedy, pp. 77-81 in *The Science of Laughter, Special TIME Edition*, Editorial Director Kostya Kennedy, New York, Time Inc. Books.

Widge AS and Miler EK (2019): Targeting cognition and networks through neural oscillation, *JAMA Psychiatry* 76(7)671-672, July 2019.

Wieder BJ et al. (2018): Wallpaper fermions and the non-symmetric Dirac insulator, *Science* 361:246-251, 20 June 2018.

Wilde L (1978): *Larry Wilde's Complete Book of Ethnic Humor*, with a Foreword by George Jessel, New York, Bell Publishing Company.

Wolfe I (2018): How a bunch of college sophomores outsmarted Princeton, Princeton, N.J., *Princeton Alumni Weekly*, March 21, 2018, p. 22.

Wolfe T(1975): *The Painted Word*, New York, Farrar, Strauss & Giroux.

Yuan L (2019): The company behind TikTok's domination, *The New York Times* Business Section, November 5, 2019, pp. B1, B7.

Ziauddeen H, Dibben C, Kipps C, Hodges JR, McKenna PJ (2010): Negative schizophrenic symptoms and the frontal lobe syndrome: one and the same? *Eur. Arch. Psychiatry Clin Neurosci* DOI:10.1107/500406-010-01-03-y 15 Aug 2010.

Zinoman J (2019): A critic's picks for the best comedy, *The New York* Times, December 25, 2019, pp. C1,C8

David V. Forrest, M.D. 155 West 68th Street, Suite 1219, New York, New York 10023; (212) 873-7750; davidvforrest@gmail.com

ABOUT THE AUTHOR

Dr. David V. Forrest

David V. Forrest, M.D. is Clinical Professor of Psychiatry and Consultant to Neurology (Movement Disorders) at Columbia University Vagelos College of Physicians & Surgeons, Past-President of The American College of Psychoanalysts, Fellow of the Explorers Club, and Founding Editor of SPRING: The Journal of the E. E. Cummings Society. He is the author of 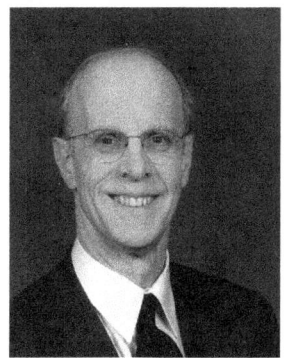 SLOTS: Praying to the God of Chance; Beyond Eden: The Other Lives of Fine Arts Models, and The Meaning of Medical Disrobing; and with his wife, Lynne Stetson, The Ballet Company Game.